THE
BELIEF
SHIFT

Rewrite Your Story. Redesign Your Life.

DENISE MOKADSI

THE BELIEF SHIFT

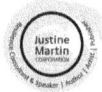

Copyright © 2025
First Published in Australia in 2025
By Morpheus Publishing PTY LTD
Geelong Victoria 3216
www.morpheuspublishing.com.au
ACN: 687 598 858 / ABN: 99687 598 858

All rights reserved. No part of this publication may be reproduced, stored in a retrieval system, or transmitted in any form or by any means, electronic, mechanical, photocopying, recording or otherwise, without the prior written permission of the publisher or author.

Paperback ISBN:	978-1-7643352-1-8
Author:	**Denise Mokadsi**
Editor:	Lynette Reurts
Cover Graphics:	Mylen Carascal

A catalogue record for this book is available from the National Library of Australia.

DISCLAIMER
The information contained in this book is for general informational purposes only. The author and publisher are not offering any medical, legal or professional advice. While every effort has been made to ensure the accuracy and completeness of the information provided, the author and publisher assume no responsibility for errors or omissions or any outcomes or consequences resulting from using this book's content.

COPYRIGHT
All original material in this book is the sole property of the author and Morpheus Publishing.

DISTRIBUTION
This book is distributed by Morpheus Publishing and is available through authorised distributors, booksellers, Morpheus Publishing website.

COPYRIGHT PERMISSIONS
For copyright permissions or any other inquiries, please contact:

PUBLISHER: Morpheus Publishing
www.morpheuspublishing.com.au | hello@morpheuspublising.com.au | +61403 564 942

AUTHOR: Denise Mokadsi https://www.morpheuspublishing.com.au/authors/denise-mokadsi

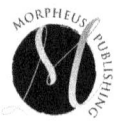

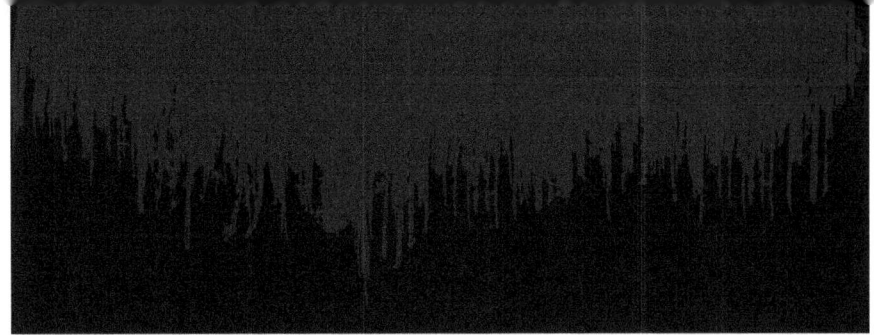

TABLE OF CONTENTS

Introduction 1

Chapter 1: The Mirror Moment 5
The Chosen Path 8
The Pull of Distraction 10
Breaking the Habit of the Overthinking Mind 12
Listening Within 13
Trusting the Unknown 15

Chapter 2: Becoming Me 19
Who Am I? 21
Who I Thought I Was 23
The Path to Identity 24
The Science of Spirituality 25
I'll Have Nun of This 26
A Deeper Sense of My Energetic Self 28

Chapter 3: A Personal Awakening 33

Below the Surface 35
Seeing Myself with New Eyes 37
Epigenetics: The Science of Influence 39
Nature and Nurture: Together as One 40
Learning from Life's Lessons 41
Finding Light in the Darkness 42
Movement as Medicine 44

Chapter 4: Generations Within Us 49

Destiny's Cradle 53
Nurturing Their Dreams, Honouring Mine 54
The Reality of Parenthood 56
Parenting the Self 57
Parenting through Consciousness 59
Awakening from the Subconscious Loop 63
Beliefs Passed Down, Beliefs Reclaimed 64
Raising an Authentic Future 66

Chapter 5: The Healing Begins 71

Becoming Your Best Healer 74
Healing from the Inside Out 76
Pain, the Unexpected Teacher 78
Living with JIA: A Lesson in Resilience 80

Listening to the Quiet Whisper 82
Turning Challenge into Opportunity 84

Chapter 6: The Blueprint Within 91
An Idea that Changed Everything 94
Unlocking the Treasure Within 97
Seeing the Whole Picture 98

Chapter 7: Staying True 103
The Everyday Mirror 105
A Family in Flow 106
Sacred Spaces of Connection 107
The Energy of Truth 108
Ordinary to Brilliant 109
Living a Real Life 111
Believe the Love You Are 112

Chapter 8: A Bigger Purpose 117
Life is the Present 120
The Power of Presence 122
The Alchemy of Desire 124
Letting Life Move Through You 125
DNA with a Purpose 126

Chapter 9: Creating What's Next 133
Disrupting the Default 136
Living by Design 138
Trusting the Slow Magic of Becoming 139
A New Path Emerging 141

Chapter 10: Integration – A Life Rewritten 147
Your Mission, if You Choose to Accept It 150
You Are Forever Changed 152
Emotion as Energy in Motion 155
Becoming the Observer of Your Life 157

Chapter 11: Not the Final Chapter, But a Living Ending 163
Seeing the Real Problem 165
Believe It. Or Not 167
No More Waiting – It's Now 170
There's Always a Good Ending 172

Gratitude and Acknowledgement 179

INTRODUCTION

I had just finished reading the final sentence and quietly laid the book down beside me. I'm often found behind the covers of a thought-provoking read, and I sensed this one would leave a lasting imprint. *Falling Down and Getting Up* by Mark Nepo had invited me to reflect on life's choices—those between surviving and thriving—and how we find inner resilience in the process. Moments from my own life began to surface, where I had stood at those same crossroads. I'm sure you've had moments like that too. Every choice we make is shaped by who we are at that point in time. And we are never quite the same person twice.

Growing up, I often heard phrases like, "If you get knocked down, get back up," or "When one door closes, another opens." They offered hope and reassurance in difficult times. Even now, as an adult navigating painful or confusing experiences, I return to those ideas. Sometimes they become transformational. Other times they're just reminders that my mindset matters. That's the motivation for this book. Because right now, as I move through a powerful midlife transition, I see the immense potential in this season of becoming. But how I move forward depends on what I believe.

The experience of my life—and the way I choose to interpret it—is mine to shape. I can stay stuck in fear, or I can open myself to love. In truth, the greatest growth often happens in the space where both meet. There's always more than one perspective to any story or situation. My work is to pause long enough to find the version of truth that is aligned with my higher self—the one rooted in love, compassion, and personal responsibility.

Optimal living isn't just about wellness and fitness. It's about creating *healthness*—an integrated experience of mind, body, and spirit. What I believe, how I feel, and the choices I make each day all shape my life. What follows in these pages is part memoir, part manual. It's the story of my personal belief shift and the strategies I've used to live more fully, more consciously, and more joyfully.

It is my hope that *The Belief Shift* offers you a fresh lens to see how your emotional history, core beliefs, and even your DNA influence the way you live. I've learned that we can rewrite the narratives we once believed were set in stone. Whether you're navigating midlife, managing a health challenge, or just sensing a deeper calling for change, this book offers insights that may guide you back to yourself.

You already have the tools. You already hold the answers. My intention is to help you remove the static that's getting in the way. You don't need to waste time doubting yourself or chasing someone else's version of success. Epigenetics has taught me that our genes are not our destiny—our lifestyle and environment play a far more powerful role. When we shift the lens through which we view the world, we change the way we experience it.

For a time, I felt overwhelmed. I was juggling a demanding family life, navigating health challenges of loved ones, and slowly burning out. Like so many women I know, I kept going—until I couldn't. Traditional advice wasn't helping. So, I turned inward and started asking different questions. Through science, holistic strategies, and inner work, I uncovered a way of living that felt authentic. I began to design my life, rather than endure it. And I've never looked back.

We all come equipped with an internal compass that can guide us back to health and wholeness. But the signals get cloudy—clouded by childhood conditioning, societal messages, outdated beliefs, and layers of self-doubt. The good news is: we can recalibrate. We can realign. And we can return to the truth of who we are.

INTRODUCTION

This book isn't about quick fixes or bypassing pain. I won't tell you how to avoid suffering or how to chase happiness. I'm here to share what I've learned about meeting life—fully, bravely, and with love. That includes the messy, uncertain parts. Especially those. Because those moments are often the doorways to transformation.

We all want to feel free, to express ourselves fully, to be seen and accepted, to grow. How we respond to life's challenges determines whether we contract in fear or expand in love. That choice lives inside us. And when we make it consciously, we step into our power.

You don't need to be fixed. You need to be reminded of who you truly are.

This is your invitation—to explore your inner world with compassion, to look at your story through a new lens, and to rediscover the strength, clarity, and creativity that have been with you all along. The path of self-awareness isn't always easy, but it is deeply rewarding. As you reflect on the questions at the end of each chapter, I hope you give yourself permission to be honest, curious, and kind.

We don't always like being knocked off our feet, but sometimes it's what we need to stand taller than before. The belief shift is not just about changing your thoughts—it's about reclaiming your power, rewriting your story, and living from the heart.

You are not the false beliefs others have placed on you—or the ones you've unknowingly absorbed. You are a conscious creator. And you are already enough.

Let's begin.

THE BELIEF SHIFT

Chapter 1
THE MIRROR MOMENT

"Wherever you are,
be there totally."

ECKHART TOLLE

I was blissfully unaware of where I was or what time it was when my 5:30 a.m. alarm shattered the stillness of sleep. Reflexively, I hit snooze and lingered in that liminal space between dreaming and waking, silently questioning why, after all these years, I was still dragging myself out of bed for early morning spin classes.

Don't get me wrong—I love a good spin session. The right playlist, a motivating instructor (which, on this particular morning, was me), and a high-energy rhythm can propel my muscles into motion. But lately, my body had been whispering in new ways—tight joints, slower recovery, a strange emotional fatigue I couldn't name. Was I just tired, or stuck in some kind of loop?

Like the film *Groundhog Day*, I noticed how easily life can become a series of repetitive, well-intentioned actions that lack true movement. Despite all the activity, something felt static. Was I really growing—or just spinning wheels?

Midlife arrives like that. Uninvited but deeply revealing. While we're guided through adolescence with whispered conversations about bras and first periods, no one really prepares us for *this*—the quieter unravelling that happens decades later. A turning inward. A reckoning. A return.

Culture urges us to stay busy, stay relevant, stay quiet. But midlife doesn't care for social scripts. It calls us toward something deeper. Not an ending—but an invitation. A soulful initiation into what comes next.

I'm proud of what I've built. Yet here I stand, at the edge of something unnamed. I'm not ready to fade quietly into the background of my own life. There are still stories to write, lessons to embody, and dreams asking to be lived. But first, I must ask: What beliefs am I still carrying? What truths have I outgrown? What parts of me have been waiting patiently to return?

Where I am today is a mosaic of every choice and experience that's come before. But the question is—where do I go from here? What story am I continuing to live? What am I willing to rewrite?

Can you relate? That quiet unrest. The inner nudge. The invisible line in the sand that marks a shift from doing to becoming. Maybe you've already begun the transformation. Maybe you're still hovering on the edge of it. Either way, you're not alone.

Like many women I know, I'm feeling the pull back to self. After decades of giving to roles and responsibilities, there's a deeper longing surfacing—a call to remember who I am beneath all the titles. What do I truly want? And what am I willing to do to live it?

As Augusten Burroughs wrote, "I am myself made entirely of flaws, stitched together with good intentions." You don't need to have it all figured out. You just need to begin with presence—with the moment you're in now.

And so we start here—with the mirror moment. The one where we pause long enough to see ourselves clearly. It may not always feel comfortable, but this kind of seeing is the beginning of real change.

We don't see the world as it is—we see it as *we* are. Through the lens of everything we've been taught, told, and taken on. Our beliefs shape what we notice, how we react, and what we think is possible.

The thing is, we rarely stop to ask *where those beliefs came from*, or whether they're even true. Most of them were formed long before we had the awareness—or the choice—to question them. And yet they quietly script the way we live.

Believe it. Or not.

Let these pages be both a mirror and a map—a gentle guide for remembering who you are and redesigning what comes next.

THE CHOSEN PATH

As a child, I loved those choose-your-own-adventure books—the kind where you made decisions for the character, flipped to a different page, and followed a new storyline. I'd read the same book multiple times, just to explore each possible ending. Looking back, it's easy to see the parallels with life: every decision creates a ripple, carving a path forward. Unlike the tidy confines of a children's book, though, real-life choices are often messy and complex.

We like to believe our lives are shaped by big decisions—the job, the house, the partner. But more often, it's the smaller, repeated choices that accumulate into a life. And those choices don't exist in a vacuum. They're shaped by who we are, the environments we live in and the levels of awareness we bring to each moment.

It's a dynamic dance—our choices shape our environment, and our environment shapes our choices. Think about it: if I live in a cold climate, I might light a fire. The resulting warmth then influences what I wear, how I feel, and even how I move through the day. This interplay is constant, subtle, and powerful. The more aware I am, the more consciously I can navigate it.

Without awareness, we default to autopilot. Our minds rely on past experiences to predict the present—sometimes usefully, other times not. We make assumptions and react out of habit. Sometimes that works. Sometimes it lands us on a metaphorical toy car in the dark.

I'll never forget one night when my kids were little. I tiptoed down the hallway for a glass of water, groggy and barefoot, only to step squarely on a sharp toy car. The pain was instant, and so was my yell—though thankfully, it didn't wake the whole house. That moment taught me something: even the most familiar path holds surprises if we walk it blindly.

Our brains crave efficiency. Habits save energy, which is great. But they also keep us repeating the same stories unless we pause and question them. When I'm reactive, I miss the opportunity to respond with intention. Awareness interrupts the loop. It brings me back to presence—and from presence, I can choose.

I can choose to see my experiences not as random events, but as invitations. I can choose to believe life is happening *for* me, not *to* me. And that choice alone transforms everything.

Mindfulness shows me where I've been—and where I have the power to go next. With it, I can piece together how the events of my life have shaped me, while also recognising that I am not defined by any single moment. Each step forward is an opportunity to respond from a new level of understanding.

Some choices have led to disappointment. Some to unexpected beauty. None of them means I'm broken. I don't need fixing—I need awareness. Acceptance. And the willingness to grow.

Healing happens when we allow it. Just as a wound heals under the right conditions, our inner hurts mend when met with care. Every moment is an opportunity to respond with love, to shift the lens, to see the experience not as punishment but as a teacher.

Sometimes, the only thing that keeps us stuck is the belief that things should be different than they are. Letting go of that resistance, even just a little, creates space for clarity, peace, and presence. And from that space, we can take the next step—one that feels aligned, grounded, and true.

THE PULL OF DISTRACTION

We live in a world that thrives on noise—constant, competing demands for our time, energy, and attention. In this fast-paced rhythm of modern life, presence becomes a practice of rebellion. It takes effort, intention, and sometimes even courage to pause, to slow down, and to truly notice where we are.

Distraction often arrives dressed as productivity. I used to believe that multitasking was the secret to efficiency—folding laundry while listening to a podcast, replying to emails while eating lunch, ticking off to-dos like I was in a race. But over time, I noticed something: the quality of my attention was thinning. The moments were blurring together. My presence was becoming diluted.

Now, I catch myself. When I'm doing the ironing, I focus on the feel of the fabric, the weight of the iron in my hand, the sound of steam, the warmth rising from the board. I notice the transformation—creases dissolving into smoothness—as a quiet metaphor for my own unfolding.

Washing dishes has become another practice. Instead of rushing through it with a podcast in the background, I notice the temperature of the water, the texture of soap bubbles, the light reflecting off the clean plates. These small rituals, once mundane, are now invitations. Anchors. Reminders to return.

Of course, I still get pulled off course. As a mother, a partner, and someone growing a business, my days are filled with demands. I've worked with coaches. I've juggled expectations. I've wrestled with self-doubt when things didn't unfold the way I hoped they would.

At times, I felt disheartened—disappointed by slow progress, frustrated by outcomes that didn't match my effort. It was tempting to chase more strategy, more doing, more fixing. But underneath that drive, I eventually found something else: a quiet but insistent belief that I wasn't enough just as I was.

That belief was the real distraction. And like most limiting beliefs, it was slippery, sneaky, and deeply ingrained.

Learning to pause—to notice the pull of distraction and question it—became a turning point. I started asking deeper questions: *"What's really driving this urgency? What am I afraid will happen if I slow down? Where am I placing my worth?"*

Gratitude has become a gentle guide. I come back to the people and moments that ground me: my family, the laughter over dinner, a morning walk, the quiet joy of watching my kids grow. In these simple moments, I remember who I am beyond the noise.

Presence isn't always easy. It takes practice. It takes forgiveness. And it requires a willingness to let go—not just of tasks, but of all the thoughts and stories that keep us spinning.

But within that pause is everything: clarity, connection, and the soft return to what truly matters.

BREAKING THE HABIT OF THE OVERTHINKING MIND

I've always been a thinker. I like figuring things out, exploring ideas from every angle, and trying to make sense of things. It's how I made it through science degrees, a nursing career, and the endless demands of motherhood and entrepreneurship. My mind has been both a faithful ally and an overzealous problem-solver. But somewhere along the way, I realised that thinking alone wasn't enough.

There came a point when the analysing, the strategising, and the mental gymnastics didn't feel empowering anymore. It felt exhausting. My head was full, but my heart felt distant. I was trying to solve problems with the same thinking that created them—looping around in familiar patterns that led to the same stuck feelings.

Einstein once said, "We cannot solve our problems with the same thinking we used when we created them." That quote hit differently when I began doing deeper inner work—when I started listening not just to my thoughts, but to what I was feeling.

Learning to let go of overthinking meant learning to trust something else—something quieter and harder to measure. It meant learning to feel more and analyse less. To sense what was right, instead of reasoning myself into or out of every decision.

Letting go didn't mean abandoning logic. It meant softening its grip. Making space for intuition. For presence. For the voice within that doesn't yell, but whispers.

When I started asking myself different questions, more helpful answers began to emerge. Not the usual *"What's wrong with me?"* but *"What might I be resisting here?"* and *"What if the solution isn't to fix this, but to feel it?"*

Often, the resistance I found was fear—fear of failure, of change, of the unknown. And though I wanted to move forward, fear kept me holding tightly to what felt safe. Even if that safety was stagnation.

Over time, I began recognising that fear wasn't something to eliminate, but something to understand. To sit with. To breathe through. And slowly, to move beyond.

This is where love entered the picture—not the romantic kind, but the energy of acceptance, compassion, and self-trust. I realised that if fear contracts, love expands. Where fear says, *"What if I can't?"*, love says, *"Let's try."*

Listening to my heart—really listening—was a new experience. It wasn't as clear-cut as following a plan. It asked more of me: stillness, vulnerability, trust. It led me back to what I'd always known deep down but had often dismissed as impractical or naive. My heart was asking to lead, not to be overridden.

And so I started practising what it meant to follow that inner guidance. To sit in meditation and wait for the whisper. To journal and let truth trickle out. To pause in the middle of the day and ask, *"What do I really need right now?"*

Sometimes the answers surprised me. Sometimes they didn't come right away. But the more I showed up, the more I realised I wasn't lost—I'd just been listening to the wrong voice.

Trusting that inner compass requires courage. It asks us to relinquish control—or at least the illusion of it. But in doing so, we open to a deeper wisdom: the quiet knowing within that connects us to something greater. Whether you call it your intuition, your higher self, or a divine intelligence, it often knows before we do.

Releasing the overthinking mind doesn't mean you stop thinking. It means your thoughts no longer run the show. Your heart begins to guide the way.

And that shift? It changes everything.

LISTENING WITHIN

One afternoon, after a meditation, I received a strong message from somewhere deep inside: follow the direction of your heart.

It was more of a knowing than a sentence. A subtle invitation, not a command. But still, questions flooded in: *"Where was this message coming from? How would I know what my heart was trying to say? Could I really trust it? Was I even listening properly?"*

In those moments, my instinct was to overthink. To spiral into analysis, plans, and pressure. But I caught myself. Breathe. Step back. Listen.

The message didn't need to be figured out. It needed to be felt.

As I tuned in, I realised there had been other times I'd followed my heart. I studied science because I loved understanding how things worked. I became a nurse because I cared deeply about people. I pursued epigenetics because I believed in the power of change. Each of these paths had meaning. Each had been guided by something more instinctual than logic.

But life has a way of pulling us off track. Responsibilities, expectations, and the endless noise of "shoulds" and "musts" can drown out that quiet voice within. Over time, I noticed I was saying yes to things that didn't feel aligned. My heart was whispering, *"This isn't it,"* but I kept going.

Eventually, I had to stop and ask myself: *"What do I really want? Why is that important to me? And what might my life look like if I honoured that truth?"*

These weren't easy questions. They required honesty and a willingness to admit where I'd been living on autopilot. But they also offered clarity—and a chance to come home to myself.

I've come to see that many women are deeply attuned to the desires of others. We're conditioned to care for, to accommodate, to anticipate. And while there's beauty in that, there's also a danger: we lose touch with our own inner voice.

Listening within doesn't mean ignoring the world. It means making space for your own wisdom to speak. It means noticing what lights you up, what drains you, what calls to you quietly but persistently. It means allowing your heart a seat at the table.

When I follow my heart, life feels richer. More honest. More meaningful. I don't always have all the answers, but I do have a compass that never fails me when I take the time to check in.

And sometimes, that's all it takes: a moment of stillness, a deep breath, and a gentle question—*"What is true for me right now?"*

That question can change your life.

TRUSTING THE UNKNOWN

Were my head and heart ever going to play nicely together—or would my overthinking mind keep trying to lead the dance? I wasn't sure. But I knew this: when I paused long enough to really listen, something softer emerged. A quieter voice. A sense of knowing without proof.

Learning to trust that voice required letting go of control, meant surrendering to the idea that I didn't need to have it all figured out. And truthfully, I never really did.

Surrender is often misunderstood. It's not about giving up. It's about loosening our grip on the outcomes we think we need and allowing life to move with us, not just around us. It's about believing that we are held—even when we don't yet understand how.

I've found this sense of trust in small but powerful moments. Like in *shavasana*, the final resting pose in yoga, when I allow my body to melt into the ground and let the earth support me. In those moments, I'm not doing anything—I'm simply being. And being, it turns out, can be the most courageous act of all.

That same principle applies to the mind. Just as we allow the body to rest in *shavasana*, we can allow the mind to rest too. To stop solving, fixing, comparing, planning. To stop measuring our worth by what we've done or what's next. To simply trust that we are supported by something greater—call it life, the universe, God, or your own inner knowing.

Our hearts already know this. The mind, however, needs convincing. It wants evidence. Guarantees. A step-by-step plan. But the heart? The heart is willing to move forward even in the fog. It whispers, *"This way"*, without needing to explain why.

Sometimes we follow that voice and the path unfolds with ease. Other times, it feels like we're walking blind. But either way, something profound happens when we choose to trust. We stop trying to control every outcome and start experiencing life as it is—raw, unpredictable, and beautiful.

Trusting the unknown doesn't mean abandoning your mind. It means allowing your heart to lead and letting your mind support that journey, not steer it.

It means finding the courage to say yes to mystery, to growth, to becoming more than who you've been.

It means believing that life will unfold with perfect timing to serve our greatest good.

And maybe that's all we ever really need: a pause long enough to ask the deeper questions. Because it's in these quiet moments of reflection that the real shifts begin. Not dramatic, not loud—but subtle, steady, sacred.

Awareness is the first act of change. It's how we reclaim our authorship. When we dare to look honestly at where we are and how we got here, we open the door to something new. Not by forcing answers, but by becoming curious observers of our own lives.

The mirror doesn't judge—it simply reflects. And in seeing ourselves more clearly, we start to soften. To realign. To recognise that we've always had more power than we believed.

This is where transformation begins—not in fixing what's wrong, but in recognising what's ready to evolve.

As we move into the next chapter, I invite you to stay close to that inner knowing. Let it guide you. Let it challenge and support you. You don't have to have it all figured out. You just have to be willing to see.

Because seeing clearly is the beginning of becoming.

Chapter Highlights

The Chosen Path:
Life is filled with choices, but choosing with presence rather than pressure allows you to align with what truly matters.

The Pull of Distraction:
Modern life thrives on urgency and noise. Reclaiming your attention is an act of self-respect.

Breaking the Habit of the Overthinking Mind:
Thought alone can't solve what the heart needs to feel. Learning to pause the mind opens space for deeper wisdom.

Listening Within:
Beneath the noise of expectation is a quiet knowing. Your heart's whisper is a compass —subtle but trustworthy.

Trusting the Unknown:
Surrendering control doesn't mean giving up. It means softening into a greater intelligence and letting life unfold one step at a time.

REFLECTIVE QUESTIONS

1. Where in your life are you choosing based on habit or pressure, rather than from presence?

2. What distracts you most easily—and what might those distractions be protecting you from feeling?

3. When was the last time you overthought something? How might you have approached it differently from the heart?

4. What signals—physical, emotional, or intuitive—let you know when you're not listening to yourself?

5. What does "trusting the unknown" mean to you right now? Is there an area of life where you could surrender just a little more?

Chapter 2
BECOMING ME

"Maybe the journey isn't about becoming anything, Maybe it's about unbecoming everything that isn't really you."

UNKNOWN

In the previous chapter, I explored some of the influences that have shaped who I am today. But as I peeled back those layers, a deeper and more intimate question began to stir: *"Who am I, really?"*

To even begin exploring this question, I had to take a step beyond familiar roles and well-worn stories. I imagined waking one morning with no memory of my name, my career, my family, or my past. If all the labels were gone—how would I recognise myself? What would be left without the scaffold of titles and responsibilities?

This is not just a philosophical question—it's a call inward. A quiet invitation to meet the version of myself that exists beyond performance and expectation. The one who was there before the world told me who to be.

In this chapter, I explore the unfolding of identity—how it's been shaped by both outer forces and inner truths, and how I'm learning to rewrite my story with more intention. As I've grown, I've come to see that identity isn't something fixed; it moves with us. It deepens, stretches, dissolves, and reforms with each new season of life.

There's a constant dance between what the world mirrors back to me and what I discover within. Family, society, work, faith—all powerful architects of the self. But so too are the quiet stirrings of my heart, my longings, my lived experience, and that still, small voice that whispers from within.

At the centre of this unfolding is a deeper essence—something that feels unchanging, even as everything else shifts. Perhaps this essence is the anchor I've been searching for. A quiet, heart-centered awareness beneath all the stories I've lived, ready to support a more meaningful and aligned way of being.

WHO AM I?

It's a question I've asked more times than I can count—sometimes in moments of stillness, other times in the middle of a personal storm.

Who am I?

It sounds so simple, yet its echo stirs something profound. What does it mean to be me?

There was a time when I believed I should have a clear, confident answer. That I should know—without hesitation—exactly who I was. But the more I've lived, the more I've realised that identity isn't a fixed statement. It's a living, breathing experience.

And maybe that's the point.

Self-discovery isn't a destination. It's not something I'll arrive at with a neat and tidy conclusion. It's a lifelong unfolding—a dance between who I've been, who I'm becoming, and the ever-changing nature of life itself. Each new experience leaves an imprint. Each chapter writes a new line in the story. And each version of myself offers a new lens through which I see the world.

Over the years, I've had to meet myself in many different forms—daughter, nurse, mother, coach, student, seeker. Some of these roles felt natural. Others were stitched together from expectation and survival. But what I've learned is that clinging too tightly to any one version of myself can keep me from growing into the next.

Identity, like the ocean, moves with the tides. Its surface may ripple with change, but beneath the waves lies something deeper—steady, still, wise.

This awareness has brought both relief and responsibility. Relief, in knowing that I don't have to stay the same to be whole. And responsibility, in learning how to meet each new version of myself with compassion and curiosity, not resistance.

One of the most powerful invitations into this kind of self-inquiry came with the transition of menopause. It unravelled long-held beliefs I'd carried about my body, my energy, my worth. The old identity no longer fit, but the new one hadn't fully formed. It felt like standing in a doorway—no longer who I was, not yet who I would become.

There were moments of discomfort, even grief. But also, a quiet strength beginning to rise.

As I surrendered to the unknown, I discovered that change doesn't have to threaten my identity—it can deepen it. When I stopped grasping and started listening, a softer, wiser self began to emerge. Not one built on roles or achievement, but on presence. On truth.

And maybe that's the answer I've been looking for all along—not a fixed definition of who I am, but a willingness to live fully in the becoming.

WHO I THOUGHT I WAS

As far back as I can remember, I've been the responsible one. The helper. The achiever. These roles weren't just descriptions—they became the framework of my identity. I wore them like well-earned badges, believing they made me valuable, lovable, and safe.

But along with these traits came a silent contract I didn't realise I'd signed. Don't fail. Don't falter. Don't stop striving. Be good. Be dependable. Be strong. I performed these roles so well, I began to forget there was ever a version of me beyond the performance.

And so, I became a version of myself shaped more by survival than by soul.

The praise I received for being helpful reinforced the behaviour. The comfort others took in my steadiness cemented the expectation. Somewhere along the way, I equated being responsible with being worthy. I confused doing with being.

But the cost of constantly holding things together—of being the one others could rely on—was that I rarely made space to consider what *I* needed. My value felt conditional. I became overly self-sufficient, afraid to ask for help, and increasingly disconnected from my own softness, vulnerability, and desires.

There's a quiet kind of grief that comes when you realise the version of you people loved was the one that needed to be strong, not the one that simply *was*.

It wasn't until I began to slow down, to ask different questions, that I noticed the gap between who I had become and who I truly was. I started to wonder: What parts of me were genuine, and what parts were carefully curated to keep me safe, accepted, or in control?

This realisation wasn't an immediate shift, but more of a gentle unfolding. A willingness to look inward, not with judgment, but with curiosity. To thank the masks I had worn for getting me through—and then slowly, lovingly, begin to take them off.

Because beneath the striving, the responsibility, and the roles, there is a self that just wants to be seen. Not for what she does, but for who she is.

THE PATH TO IDENTITY

Identity isn't something we're born fully knowing—it's something we inherit, absorb, question, and ultimately, choose.

As I began to peel back the layers of who I thought I was, I noticed how many of those layers were borrowed. Some were lovingly handed down by family. Others were shaped by cultural messages, religion, education, or the quiet need to fit in. These external influences had formed a kind of scaffolding around my sense of self. They gave me structure and belonging—but they also created limits.

There came a point when the identity I had carefully constructed started to feel more like a costume than a second skin. I felt hemmed in, like I was living within the blueprint of someone else's design. But stepping out of that blueprint required something terrifying and beautiful: the courage to not know who I was for a little while.

At first, I tried to hold on to the familiar. I kept performing roles that once earned me approval. I tried to fit back into old identities like jeans that no longer hugged in the right places. But eventually, discomfort became the invitation to grow. The cracks in my self-image became the spaces where light began to shine through.

I realised that while I had inherited many parts of my identity, I was not obligated to keep them all. Some pieces were outgrown. Others never truly fit. And some, when examined closely, were never mine to carry.

That awareness created space. Space to pause. To ask, *"Who am I, really—and who do I want to be now?"*

The journey didn't give me a final answer. What it gave me was something far more valuable: permission. Permission to evolve. To edit my story. To choose again.

And so, identity became less about fixing who I am, and more about flowing with who I am becoming.

THE SCIENCE OF SPIRITUALITY

For as long as I can remember, I've been drawn to understanding how things work. Science gave me a language to make sense of the world—logical, structured, and evidence-based. It provided answers, or at the very least, frameworks to explore them. As a nurse and lifelong learner, I was trained to observe symptoms, identify patterns, and rely on what could be measured and tested.

And yet, somewhere along the way, I began to notice what couldn't be measured—those moments that defied logic but felt undeniably true.

I'd sense something before it happened. I'd walk into a room and feel a shift in energy without a word being spoken. I'd experience quiet inner knowings that offered more clarity than any textbook ever could. These experiences didn't fit neatly into scientific categories, but they were real to me.

There was a time I felt hesitant to admit this. I didn't want to appear irrational or "woo-woo". But I also couldn't ignore the gentle tug of curiosity that invited me into a deeper exploration of something less tangible but equally powerful.

I found myself at a bridge between two worlds—one rooted in science, the other in spirituality. I didn't want to choose one over the other. I wanted to hold both. To trust the data and still honour the divine. To acknowledge the brilliance of biology while embracing the mystery of consciousness.

Science explains the *how*. Spirituality explores the *why*. When brought together, they reveal something more whole.

As I studied epigenetics, I saw how beliefs, environment, and mindset could influence gene expression. This wasn't mystical thinking—it was the science of how our inner and outer worlds shape our biology. The line between matter and meaning began to blur in the most beautiful way.

There's a richness in holding both logic and intuition. One grounds me, the other uplifts me. Together, they have helped me reclaim a fuller, more expansive understanding of who I am—not just a physical body, but an energetic, emotional, and spiritual being, too.

I'LL HAVE NUN OF THIS

Not everyone reading this book will have a connection to religion, faith, or spirituality—and that's okay. But for me, it was always going to be part of my story. From the earliest moments of my life, even before I took my first breath, the seeds of faith had already been sown.

Before my parents met, my mother had chosen a different path—one deeply rooted in devotion. Raised in a devout Catholic family as the sixth child of ten, she felt an early and powerful calling to religious life. In her early twenties, she entered a convent and began training to become a nun. Her days were filled with prayer, service, and contemplation. She explored the vows of poverty, chastity, and obedience with sincerity, fully intending to dedicate her life to God.

But just before taking her final vows, something shifted. A quiet knowing stirred within her—this wasn't her path after all. She left the convent, unsure of what lay ahead, but certain she had to trust the nudge. Not long after, she met my father. He likes to joke that somehow he was the reason she changed her mind, even though they hadn't yet met. Maybe he was right. The universe often works in mysterious ways.

Though she left the convent, her faith never left her. It remained a guiding force in her life and, naturally, became part of mine too.

I grew up in a home where Catholicism wasn't just a religion—it was a way of life. Sunday Mass, prayers before meals and before going to sleep, saint icons on the walls, and a quiet reverence woven into the everyday. The rituals were familiar, comforting even. They created structure and a sense of belonging. Community, care, and tradition were the steady undercurrent of my childhood.

I admired the nuns at my school—their grace, their certainty, their unwavering devotion. There was something magnetic about them. And yet, beneath their poise, I felt a quiet tension rise in me. I had questions—questions about God, about suffering, about the contradictions I sensed between what was taught and what I instinctively felt to be true. Why was God to be feared? Why did questioning feel like rebellion? Why did faith sometimes require us to silence what we intuitively knew?

I was a curious child—eager not just to believe, but to understand. But sometimes curiosity could look a lot like disobedience. So I learned to quiet my questions, to be the good girl, to nod along even when something in me didn't quite fit.

Still, those questions never left. They simply went quiet until I was old enough—and brave enough—to hear them again.

While the routine has changed somewhat now, spirituality has replaced organised religion. Doing so wasn't a rejection of faith. It was an act of honesty. Spirituality became less about rituals and more about relationship. Less about dogma, more about direct experience. I wasn't turning my back on faith—I was walking towards a truer one.

My conversations with the divine are now quiet and daily. They happen in nature, in stillness, in the moments I pause long enough to listen. My own personal relationship validates the connection. I trust the quiet wisdom within to guide me.

Looking back, I see how my mother's journey shaped my own—not in the path she walked, but in her courage to listen when the call changed. Her decision to leave the convent wasn't the end of her faith—it was the beginning of a new, more authentic chapter. And the same became true for me.

A DEEPER SENSE OF MY ENERGETIC SELF

As I've grown in awareness, I've come to realise that my identity isn't just shaped by the mind or the stories I carry—but by something more subtle, more embodied: energy.

Not the kind you measure with kilojoules or track with a fitness app, but the kind you feel. The kind that shifts a room when someone walks in. The kind that tells you, without words, whether you're safe, seen, or stifled. The kind that either drains you or lights you up.

I used to override this energetic awareness. I'd power through fatigue, people-please my way through discomfort, and make choices that looked good on paper but felt heavy in my body. I mistook productivity for purpose. I didn't yet understand that energy holds its own intelligence—and that learning to listen to it would become one of my most powerful tools for transformation.

Now, I pay attention. I notice the sensations in my body when something is aligned—or when it's not. I notice which environments help me breathe more deeply and which ones cause me to shrink. I've learned to ask myself: Am I doing this out of obligation or inspiration? Is this energising or depleting? Am I expanding or contracting?

Practices like breathwork, movement, meditation, and grounding have helped me reconnect with this intuitive wisdom. They remind me that presence isn't just a mindset—it's a vibration. A felt sense of being at home in myself.

This awareness has also helped me see others more clearly. I can sense when someone's words don't match their energy, or when they're carrying a weight they haven't named. It's given me more compassion and a deeper appreciation for the unspoken language we all share.

As I continue this journey, I've come to believe that our energetic signature—the way we feel to ourselves and to others—is one of the truest expressions of who we are. When we honour and nurture that energy, we return to a more authentic, grounded, and aligned version of ourselves.

And perhaps, at the core of it all, this is the real self I've been searching for—not a fixed identity, but a living frequency. One that is quiet, clear, and connected.

It doesn't need a title or a role. It simply is.

This deeper self doesn't shout. It doesn't strive. It gently guides, like a compass pointing home. And as I learn to listen, I realise that becoming isn't about becoming someone else—it's about returning to the truth of who I've always been.

The journey of becoming me isn't linear. It's layered. Ongoing and alive. And it begins by softening the grip on who I thought I had to be—so I can finally become who I already am.

Chapter Highlights

Who Am I?:
Identity isn't something we find—it's something we continually create.

Who I Thought I Was:
The roles we play in childhood can become masks we forget we're wearing.

The Path to Identity:
Letting go of outdated self-images shaped by inherited beliefs opens space for curiosity, renewal, and a more soul-aligned version of self.

The Science of Spirituality:
True understanding is found not in choosing between logic and intuition, but in learning how to listen to both.

I'll Have Nun of This:
Questioning dogma is not rebellion—it's often the beginning of an authentic spiritual journey.

A Deeper Sense of My Energetic Self:
Reconnecting with our energetic body allows for a more embodied, present, and intuitive way of living.

REFLECTIVE QUESTIONS

1. In this season of your life, what feels true about who you are—and what no longer fits?
   _____
   _____

2. What labels or expectations from childhood still shape how you show up today?
   _____
   _____

3. Where might you be holding on to outdated versions of yourself out of familiarity, fear, or loyalty?
   _____
   _____

4. In what ways can you honour both your analytical mind and your intuitive heart?
   _____
   _____

5. What early beliefs about faith or authority are you ready to re-examine or release?
   _____
   _____

6. How does your energy guide you toward truth or away from alignment—and are you willing to trust it more fully?
   _____
   _____
   _____

THE BELIEF SHIFT

Chapter 3

A PERSONAL AWAKENING

"Knowing yourself is the beginning of all wisdom."

ARISTOTLE

By the time midlife arrived, I had mastered the art of managing, achieving, and keeping it all together. From the outside, it probably looked like I was thriving. But inwardly, something had begun to unravel—quietly, insistently.

It wasn't a lightning bolt moment. No dramatic crisis or breakdown. Just a series of subtle but undeniable signals: persistent fatigue, physical symptoms I couldn't explain, a restlessness I couldn't name. It was as if a deeper part of me had been whispering for years, and I'd finally paused long enough to hear it.

That whisper wasn't asking me to fix myself. It was asking me to *remember* who I was beneath all the roles and responsibilities I'd accumulated. This was the start of my personal awakening—not a single event, but a slow, sacred return to myself.

This chapter is about that awakening. The moment I began to understand that living a full life isn't just about what we achieve or produce—it's about how deeply we know ourselves. Not the version curated for others, but the one grounded in inner truth. In values. In the quiet wisdom that lives beneath the noise.

Awakening doesn't always arrive wrapped in light. More often, it begins in shadow—with discomfort, confusion, and grief for the self we're outgrowing. But in that vulnerable space, something essential begins to stir. Something real. Something free.

BELOW THE SURFACE

From the outside, my life looked fine—good even. A career in health, a busy family life, and all the right things in place. But beneath the surface, I was beginning to unravel.

I didn't notice it all at once. It came in waves—trouble sleeping, an undercurrent of irritability, and a persistent feeling that something was missing.

At first, I chalked it up to stress or hormones. But the more I tried to push through, the more I felt out of alignment with myself.

Adding more fuel to the fire, the local gyms that I worked at were all shut down. Experiencing several of the longest lockdowns in the world, I was presented with an opportunity to completely change the way I was spending my time.

There's a quote I've heard many times: "When the student is ready, the teacher appears", often attributed to Lao Tzu. While the origins of this quote may be a little unclear, I've come to see its truth in my own life. Sometimes the teacher is a person. Other times, it's a moment, a challenge, or a quiet nudge from within. In this case, it came through a sudden change in my employment.

Finding myself on "forced leave", I knew this was the perfect time for me to quench my growing curiosity about why we behave the way we do, what drives our thoughts, our health, our habits, and even our inertia–what keeps us stuck.

That curiosity led me to enrol in an epigenetics health coaching course. What I discovered there completely transformed how I see myself, my health, and the way I navigate the world.

Understanding the core ingredients of the "Denise recipe" meant asking deeper questions. At times that felt confronting, but curiosity can be a powerful companion to courage. Directing light into dark corners can prove there is nothing to be afraid of.

I began to wonder: How much of my life experience is the result of my biology, and how much is shaped by my environment? How do all these elements interact?

That's when I realised: personal awakening is not a single moment. It's an ongoing return to self-understanding and self-acceptance. Self-awareness shines a light on hidden limiting beliefs. Self-compassion helps me make peace with their presence—so I can gently begin to let them go.

This realisation didn't come with instant clarity or a five-step plan. It came with a decision to stop ignoring myself and come home to the real ME.

It's about recognising my desires, releasing the resistance, forgiving myself for believing the non-truths, and choosing to expand instead. Expansion, for me, means showing up more fully, more honestly, and more meaningfully, in ways that connect with others as we share this life experience together.

We want to belong. We want to survive. But we create stories—not just about situations, but about who we are—that help us feel secure in our place within the tribe.

What happens when those stories keep us small? When does the false story become the one we believe? And to what extent does it affect our other stories about who we believe we are? What must we be willing to see, question, or shift in order to come back to who we really are?

SEEING MYSELF WITH NEW EYES

As I began to peel back the layers of my busy, outwardly "together" life, I started to notice how much of my identity had been built around what I could do for others. Being capable, reliable, efficient—these were the traits that earned praise, trust, and a sense of belonging. They were the foundation of my self-worth. But they also became a mask.

This mask of capability was useful. It helped me thrive in work and keep my family running. It allowed me to be the dependable one, the strong one, the one who didn't fall apart. But beneath it, I often felt unseen and emotionally distant—even from myself.

Midlife has a way of handing us a mirror, one that doesn't just reflect how others see us, but how we've come to see ourselves. And what I saw in that mirror was a woman who had learned to wear strength like armour, often at the expense of her own needs, softness, and self-trust.

There was a moment—I remember it clearly—when someone asked me, "What do you need right now?" And I didn't know how to answer. I had spent so long tuning into everyone else's needs that I had lost the ability to hear my own.

This was the lens I had been seeing life through: productivity over presence, doing over being, performance over authenticity.

The realisation didn't feel shameful—it felt liberating. Because once we can see the lens, we can change it. I began to ask myself different questions: *"What lights me up? What drains me? When do I feel most alive?"*

Slowly, I started to reclaim parts of myself I had tucked away. Creative parts. Restful parts. Curious parts. I didn't need to abandon the capable woman I had been—I just needed to change the lens through which I saw myself. It wasn't about fixing who I was—it was about rediscovering who I had always been, underneath the noise.

Epigenetics opened my eyes to the intricate and holistic nature of our human experience. I began to understand how our thoughts, feelings, and behaviours are shaped, not just by our upbringing or our environment, but also by our biology. It became clear to me that we need to consider both nature *and* nurture if we want to support our wellbeing in a sustainable and empowered way.

What I found was more than just science. It was an exciting new view of myself.

It helped me see myself more clearly and without judgment. I began to understand the "why" behind many of my patterns: my beliefs, values, preferences, biases, and even some of the invisible rules I'd been living by without realising it.

This new awareness gave me something profound. It gave me permission to be myself. And, more than that, it gave me the tools to consciously shape the outcomes I desired. It was the kind of knowledge that doesn't just inform, it liberates.

One of my most powerful insights was this: by the time we're old enough to question the stories we've been told, we're already seeing the world through a lens shaped by those very stories. Even the *act* of questioning is coloured by what we've absorbed over time. It reminded me of wearing a pair of tinted glasses and forgetting they were even on—until someone points it out. The lenses we wear shape what we see, how we interpret it, and what we believe is possible.

And still, with awareness, we can choose to take them off, or at the very least, clean off the smudges.

Our unique makeup—through genetics and lifestyle—means that no two people experience life in the same way. What one person finds overwhelming, another might see as effortless. That made me pause. *Much of my experience was shaped by my perception of that experience.*

Epigenetics gave me the framework to explore how I perceived the world. It showed me that I have more influence in the unfolding of my identity, my choices and potential than I ever imagined. It helped me see myself with new eyes. And once you've seen through that lens, there's no going back.

EPIGENETICS: THE SCIENCE OF INFLUENCE

Epigenetics may not be a term everyone is familiar with, but its message is profoundly empowering: we are not bound by our genes. While our DNA sequence is set from birth, the way those genes express themselves over time can change—dramatically—based on the lives we lead.

The word "epigenetics" literally means "above the genes". It refers to the study of how environmental factors—like stress, sleep, diet, exercise, relationships, and mindset—can switch genes on or off, influencing how they function without changing the DNA itself.

This explains how two people with the same genetic blueprint (like identical twins) can have entirely different health outcomes. One person may develop a condition while the other does not—not because their genes are different, but because their environments and lifestyles influence which genes are activated.

That idea felt revolutionary to me. Suddenly, I wasn't just at the mercy of my biology. I had a say. I had agency. My daily choices—how I moved, how I ate, how I rested, how I responded to stress—weren't just about willpower or discipline. They were shaping my future at a cellular level.

It also made me curious: how much of my behaviour was shaped by my genes, and how much by the environment I had grown up in?

Did my early life stressors, family dynamics, cultural expectations, or genetics play a role in the patterns I struggled to break?

The answer, of course, is yes. Both nature and nurture matter. Our genetic code may write the script, but it's the epigenetic signals that decide which scenes get played. Our DNA is the blueprint—but our environment holds the pen.

That realisation invited me to reframe my self-awareness journey. I began to see myself not just through the lens of personality or past experiences, but through a wider view: one that honoured both the science of my biology and the wisdom of my life choices.

And from that place a more hopeful truth emerged: change is possible. Healing is possible. Not by becoming someone new, but by supporting the version of me that's already there waiting to be expressed more fully.

NATURE AND NURTURE: TOGETHER AS ONE

It's no coincidence that I am where I am and who I am today. Every step—every joy, every struggle—has shaped the woman I've become. My genes and my environment aren't opposing forces; they're dance partners, moving together to influence every aspect of my development.

And that's not just poetic—it's biological.

When I completed my own epigenetic assessment, I discovered my unique body type was predominantly shaped by the mesoderm—the middle embryonic germ layer formed early in development. All of us are formed from three of these foundational layers: the endoderm, ectoderm, and mesoderm. Each one plays a crucial role in building the architecture of our body, influencing everything from organ systems to energy patterns.

The endoderm gives rise to the inner linings of our digestive and respiratory systems, as well as organs like the liver and pancreas. The ectoderm forms the skin, brain, and nervous system. And the mesoderm—my dominant type—contributes to the development of muscles, bones, connective tissues, blood vessels, kidneys, the heart, and the adrenal cortex.

Awareness of this mesodermal influence brought a new understanding of myself. People with this type often have a naturally athletic frame and a strong drive, thanks to heightened adrenal function and hormones like testosterone. Traits such as leadership, persistence, and courage were familiar to me—but so were the downsides: reactivity, intensity, and self-judgment.

By the time I reached my 50s, I thought I had a pretty good grasp on who I was. But epigenetics offered a deeper perspective—one that helped explain why I responded to life the way I did. It was like someone had handed me the manual I didn't know I was missing.

There was comfort in that clarity—and a quiet grief, too. I grieved for the years I spent trying to change parts of myself that were never broken, just misunderstood. And I felt comfort in seeing myself more clearly, more compassionately, through this new lens.

It all began to make sense. The parts of me I had tried to tame or push away were often aligned with my natural blueprint. And when I tried to override those instincts, it felt like swimming against the current of who I truly was.

Understanding this didn't limit me—it freed me. It gave me permission to be more fully myself and to operate from my natural strengths with confidence instead of apology.

Because self-awareness isn't about fixing who we are, it's about seeing and accepting who we've always been.

LEARNING FROM LIFE'S LESSONS

Awareness of how certain situations affect me has become one of the most valuable tools I carry. Through a more compassionate lens, I've learned to recognise that my responses—whether thoughtful or reactive—are often just my inner and outer worlds trying to talk to each other.

I now understand more clearly the reasons behind my habits, my emotions, and even the ways I move through a day or communicate under pressure. That understanding brings choice. It softens the edges of self-judgement and opens the door to gentler growth.

Life remains a work in progress. The messy parts, the rushed mornings, the moments when I still forget to breathe—these are not signs of failure. They are invitations to bring more presence into my choices. The more I pay attention, the more skilful I become at creating outcomes that reflect who I want to be.

I don't always get it right. Like the time I was rushing between tasks as a working mum, trying to return some party equipment in the middle of a rainy day. The traffic was slow, I didn't know the area well, and instead of trusting the car's navigation, I took a "shortcut" that delayed me even more. I ended up arriving late, parked too quickly, missed the small print on a sign, and came back to a ticket on my windscreen.

That frustrating moment wasn't just about bad luck. It was a product of my patterns of behaviour—the rushing, overriding my own limits, trying to be efficient at all costs.

When we're willing to look closely, these everyday experiences become our greatest teachers. They reveal the beliefs we've outgrown, the behaviours that drain us, and the places where we can choose differently.

And that's the gift. We can always choose again. With awareness, we gain the freedom to evolve, the freedom to shift our beliefs.

Not by becoming someone new, but by slowly, lovingly, becoming more ourselves.

FINDING LIGHT IN THE DARKNESS

When I think back to my childhood, I remember often feeling defensive and reactive. My default was to brace for impact. I didn't always understand where those reactions came from, but they became familiar, automatic responses that led to conflict, avoidance, or shutdown. What I know now is that for better outcomes, we need better behaviour. And for better behaviour, we need a belief shift that comes from deeper self-awareness.

It starts with the willingness to look at what we usually hide from ourselves.

When we shine a compassionate light on our less helpful behaviours, we can begin to identify the limiting beliefs that quietly drive them. These beliefs, things like *"I'm not good enough"* or *"I'm not worthy"*, create a cascade of internal consequences. They distort our thoughts, generate low-energy emotions, and trigger behaviours that keep us stuck. They aren't just mental patterns; they become part of us. And over time, they shape our identity, not because they're true—but because we believe them.

One of the biggest breakthroughs for me was understanding that my biology also plays a role in this patterning. My genetic makeup, especially my body's relationship to adrenaline, influences how I react, whether under stress or not. A mesomorphic body with higher sensitivity to adrenaline will respond with more intensity. For me, that often showed up as a desire to act—to *do* something, *fix* something, or *fight* something.

Knowing this doesn't excuse the behaviour, but it explains it. And that's empowering.

For me, limiting beliefs tend to provoke an "attack" response. The moment I feel criticised or misunderstood, my biology nudges me to defend myself. Those triggers used to happen without pause—but now, with awareness, I can step into a more conscious response. I've learned to meet those moments with curiosity rather than blame, and to ask: *"What if this isn't about me being flawed? What if this is just how my body protects me?"*

That simple reframing helps me soften. I no longer see my reactivity as something to shame, but as a signal. A signpost. An opportunity to pause, breathe, and choose a new way.

Now when I feel that familiar heat rise—when I sense the urge to fight back—I stop and ask myself: *"What can I do here instead of attacking? What if I don't need to defend myself right now? How would I respond then?"*

Just asking the question opens the space I need to step out of old patterns and into a more grounded, self-compassionate response. I am able to be both kinder to myself and to others. Because the truth is, the light was always there. I just needed to stop hiding from it.

MOVEMENT AS MEDICINE

Understanding my biology has revealed to me just how essential and powerful movement is for me—not just as a habit, but as a lifeline. Even as a child, I was always in motion—dribbling basketballs, riding bikes, chasing tennis balls, sprinting through netball drills. My parents often joked that I never sat still, and in hindsight, they weren't wrong.

What I understand clearly now is that I didn't just *enjoy* movement—I *needed* it. Movement has always been a way for me to regulate, to release, and to return to myself. It helps me discharge adrenaline, process emotion, and reconnect with my body's rhythm. When I go too long without it, I start to feel stagnant, short-tempered, and disconnected.

That's the mesodermal blueprint at work. With a naturally high sensitivity to adrenaline, my body thrives on movement—it's how I metabolise stress and stay grounded. This wasn't just about being sporty as a kid. It was, and still is, about energy flow. About emotional processing. About staying balanced in a fast-moving world.

Today, this understanding helps me plan my life with more self-awareness. It means knowing that my biology and environment aren't obstacles—they're allies. I know I function best in the morning when my energy is high. I know that daily movement—whether it's a walk, a stretch, or something more intense—is not optional for me. It's vital. And I know that my assertiveness or restlessness in high-pressure situations isn't a flaw—it's how I'm wired.

This knowledge has quieted the inner critic. It's given me permission to work *with* my nature instead of against it. To honour the signals my body sends, and to choose self-support over self-judgement.

Movement is no longer something I fit in around the edges of my day—it's something I build my day around. Because when I move my body, I move through emotion, restore clarity, and return to myself.

It's not just exercise. For me, it's medicine.

This chapter documents a personal awakening—an invitation to meet myself with fresh eyes. By honouring the interplay between my biology and my lived experiences, I've begun to see myself not as a puzzle to fix, but as a story to understand. A story shaped by both nature and nurture, yet always open to rewriting.

Awakening isn't a single moment. It's a process of remembering. Of noticing what no longer fits and gently turning toward what does. It asks us to listen more closely—to the body, to intuition, to the quiet wisdom that's been there all along.

So I ask you: What might your personal awakening look like? Where is life asking you to pay attention? And are you willing to pause long enough to truly hear the answer?

Chapter Highlights

Below the Surface:
Self-awareness begins when we question the stories we've believed, confront the discomfort of change, and choose to come home to our real selves.

Seeing Myself with New Eyes:
True transformation begins with the courage to see ourselves differently—not as flawed, but as evolving.

Epigenetics: The Science of Influence:
Our genes are not our destiny. Epigenetics shows us that our environment, beliefs, and behaviours shape how our genes express themselves.

Nature and Nurture: Together as One:
Who we are is formed by both our biology and our experiences—each playing a vital role in shaping our identity.

Learning from Life's Lessons:
Everyday challenges reflect the habits and patterns that need our attention. With curiosity, they become powerful opportunities for growth.

Finding Light in the Darkness:
Limiting beliefs, often formed in childhood, can become embodied patterns that shape our adult responses.

Movement as Medicine:
Understanding the biology behind our needs helps us live in alignment with our natural rhythms.

REFLECTIVE QUESTIONS

1. Where in your life do you find yourself reacting automatically, and what might those reactions be trying to protect?
   _____
   _____
   _____

2. Can you recall a time when greater self-awareness helped you make a different choice? What was the outcome?
   _____
   _____
   _____

3. How does understanding the role of both nature and nurture shift the way you view your personal challenges?
   _____
   _____
   _____

4. What would it look like to meet yourself with more compassion and curiosity in moments of discomfort or defence?
   _____
   _____
   _____

5. What inner gifts are you beginning to see more clearly as you understand yourself more deeply?
   _____
   _____
   _____

THE BELIEF SHIFT

Chapter 4

GENERATIONS WITHIN US

"No legacy is so rich as honesty."
"This above all: to thine own self be true, and it must follow as the night the day, thou canst not then be false to any man."

WILLIAM SHAKESPEARE

In the timeless words of Shakespeare, we're reminded that truth begins with self-honesty. This idea echoes the findings of Bronnie Ware, author of *The Top Five Regrets of the Dying*, who found that many people's greatest regret at the end of life was not having lived true to themselves.

Earlier chapters explored the many forces that shape our identity—our biology, our upbringing, and our beliefs. But no experience brought this into clearer focus for me than becoming a parent. In trying to raise children with a sense of confidence and self-worth, I was confronted with a deeper truth: I could not ask them to be authentic if I was not willing to be honest with myself.

Parenting shone a light on the legacy I was creating—not just through the things I said, but through who I was being. The values I inherited from my own parents—their fears, strengths, and silent expectations—had shaped me more than I realised. And now, I could see those threads beginning to weave into the lives of my children.

This realisation was both humbling and empowering.

Our children may hear our words, but they learn from our actions. They sense our energy, feel our tension, and absorb our beliefs. If I wanted my children to feel safe being themselves, I needed to model that safety through my own presence, vulnerability, and truth.

I remember one particular afternoon with my son. He'd had a rough day at school—he was withdrawn, frustrated, and unsure of himself. My instinct was to offer advice or share my own story to make him feel better. But something told me to pause. Instead, I asked him gently, "What do you need right now?"

He looked at me and said, "I just need to know it's okay to feel like this."

That moment stayed with me. Not because I got it right, but because I finally understood: he didn't need fixing. He needed space. He needed someone to trust his process.

It was a turning point. I realised that my role as a parent wasn't to shape him into who I thought he should be—it was to support him in becoming who he already is.

Children aren't here to relive our lives. They're here to live their own.

To support them in doing that, we must look inward. Parenting asks us to revisit the beliefs we absorbed in childhood: Is love something I must earn? Is vulnerability safe? Am I only worthy when I achieve?

These questions often live just below the surface, passed down not through conscious intent, but through quiet repetition. But once seen, they can be interrupted. This is the moment of the Belief Shift: when we become aware of what we've inherited and choose to shift the narrative.

Because what we don't transform, we transmit.

And what we choose to transform becomes the new legacy.

This process is not about being perfect. It's about being present. Our presence is what creates the environment in which new beliefs can take root—not just for ourselves, but for the generations that follow.

As I reflect on my own upbringing, I see now how much I internalised simply by watching my parents move through the world. Their beliefs—spoken and unspoken—became the lens through which I saw myself. And without realising it, I began to pass those same patterns on.

The invitation of this chapter is a gentle one: to pause and look inward. To become curious about the beliefs we carry, the ones we inherited, and the ones we're choosing—perhaps unknowingly—to pass along.

Legacy isn't just about what we leave behind. It's about how we show up now.

With greater self-awareness, we gain greater choice. And in that choice is the power to shift everything.

We can't change the past. But we can shift the story. We can choose presence over perfection. Courage over fear. And truth over legacy left unexamined.

Because when we shift a belief, we shift a lineage.

DESTINY'S CRADLE

From my earliest years, the idea of nurturing life held a deep resonance within me. As a child, I was playful and curious, embracing each new experience without the tangled overthinking that often burdens adults.

At the age of two, my world expanded when a new playmate—a little sister—joined our family. Though memories of that time are mostly glimpses and snapshots, our family photo album tells the story of a big sister gently watching over her little companion, sharing bath times, meals, playtimes, and all the quiet moments in between.

Those early years were filled with morning tea parties, afternoons swinging in the backyard, splashing in a small inflatable pool on warm evenings, bike rides, hopscotch, doll prams, and the simple joy of heading off to school hand-in-hand.

Seven years later, the arrival of twin sisters brought even more life and laughter. For my father, it meant "more mouths to feed", but for me, it was an invitation to deeper connection and nurturing, weaving a shared life journey with these special souls.

Life, of course, is never static. New homes, new schools, and new friends marked chapters in my evolving story, but through it all, a steady foundation of parental love and guidance remained. The family values instilled in us—love, respect, honesty, openness, empathy, positivity, communication, problem-solving, safety, resilience, and kindness—were the pillars that shaped not just our personalities but the very fabric of our relationships. These values have endured, especially when life's inevitable challenges have tested them over time.

Beyond the family, the developing brain plays a vital role in shaping a young identity. Each of us responds to life's circumstances in unique ways—our perspectives, emotions, and behaviours are personal and varied, even between identical twins. This complexity arises from an intricate dance between our genetics, the love and care we receive, the meanings we assign to our experiences, and the many environmental factors that shape us. Our lives unfold as expressions of this rich interplay.

As a young child, much of this shaping happened without conscious awareness. Like a sponge, my mind absorbed everything around me, forming impressions and beliefs that ranged from positive to painful.

For instance, I quickly learned that crying when hungry brought food and comfort; this simple association between inner need and outer response formed an early bridge between myself and the world. But I also learned lessons of caution. I remember the searing heat of a hot pavement on a barefoot summer day, teaching me to associate certain experiences with pain and avoidance.

Every habit and belief programmed in childhood shapes and directs us. Some help us thrive; others no longer serve us. As an adult, I face the profound task of unlearning those hidden subconscious patterns that limit me and consciously rewriting the programming to align with who I truly want to be.

This ongoing process of awareness, release, and transformation is at the heart of The Belief Shift—the journey toward becoming the fullest, most authentic version of ourselves. I will explore this powerful work further in the chapters ahead.

NURTURING THEIR DREAMS, HONOURING MINE

As I continued to weave my own tapestry through time, I felt a strong pull toward the specialised world of neonatal intensive care. The Neonatal Intensive Care Unit (NICU) is a high-pressure environment where premature or critically ill newborns receive continuous medical and nursing care. Working alongside neonatologists and allied health professionals, I found deep meaning in this work—physically, mentally, emotionally, and spiritually.

It was a privilege to walk beside families in their most vulnerable moments.

And experiencing this calling before becoming a mother myself gave me a front-row seat to one of life's most powerful relationships: the bond between parent and child.

Whether this yearning came from my upbringing, my natural inner strengths, or a combination of both, I had always felt a deep desire to become a mother. Over time, I noticed a recurring pattern in my life: when I truly decide something—when I align my thoughts, feelings, and actions—a series of opportunities often begins to unfold. It's as though the decision itself sets the wheels in motion.

After completing postgraduate studies in neonatal nursing, marrying my partner, and settling into our first home, the next natural step was imagining a family of our own.

At the time, I was working as a nurse unit manager in a tertiary teaching hospital. The role came with a steep learning curve: coordinating a 30-bed unit and leading a team of over 250 staff. It was demanding and fulfilling, but also stressful. I constantly felt the need to perform, to do it all just right. Looking back, much of that pressure came from within—fuelled by perfectionism and a strong internal drive.

Despite every test showing "nothing wrong," conceiving a child wasn't as straightforward as I'd hoped. The stress from work began to spill into other areas of life, and I wondered whether something beyond my control was at play.

Then, quietly and unexpectedly, a new opportunity arose. I accepted a role as a neonatal nurse educator at the Royal Children's Hospital in Melbourne. It felt like the right fit—a chance to honour my clinical expertise, embrace my love of teaching, and find a more balanced rhythm.

I still remember the morning of the interview. I felt calm and aligned. On my way in, I bumped into a former colleague whose friendly chat reinforced my sense of belonging. By the time I sat down with the interview panel, I felt present and connected. It was as if everything had aligned.

What I didn't expect was that this new professional path would open the door to a long-awaited personal dream. With the shift in pace, the easing of pressure, and the joy of doing what I loved, something within me softened. And with that softening, something beautiful took root.

A long-held hope literally began to bloom. A dream I had carried quietly for years was finally ready to be born.

THE REALITY OF PARENTHOOD

With a baby on the way, I thought: Now the real work begins. I had years of experience with sick babies, so surely a healthy baby would be a whole lot easier, or at least, that's what I told myself. But parenting is a whole different ball game when you're the one on the court.

The transition from the theoretical realm of parenting books and prenatal classes to the tangible, lived experience was transformative. As parents, we bear witness to the unfolding of a tiny life, delicate yet resilient. The weight of responsibility presses down with significant force—a responsibility to guide, nurture, and help shape a future identity.

There was going to be a new little person joining our family. What would they be like? What kind of parents would we be? How would we bond together as mother and child, and as a new family unit? What did life have in store for us? It was a time filled with both excitement and hesitation.

Before stepping fully into my new role as a mother, I found myself reflecting on how my own childhood experiences might influence the kind of parent I would become. The attachments formed in my earliest years set the groundwork for the relationships I built later in life. I learned about connection by watching the interactions of those closest to me. I learned how to feel about my body by observing how my parents felt about theirs. I learned how to relate to money by watching their relationship with it. I learned how to prioritise self-care by witnessing whether they did. I learned how to respond to challenges by watching their responses.

As an impressionable young child, I relied on my primary caregivers to keep me safe, to offer guidance, and to model what life looked like. I mirrored their behaviours in an attempt to learn how to engage with the world. Their reality shaped my reality. And amid the sleepless nights, cries, and first steps of my own children, the profound truth that this would be true for them too hit home. I was now the mirror.

As a parent, I hold significant influence over my children, and I need to stay conscious of that influence. I don't believe there is a greater responsibility. This awareness is especially crucial during the early, impressionable years of their identity development. My behaviour is their blueprint. My internal state influences the tone of our interactions, the safety of our connection, and the stories they begin to tell themselves about who they are.

PARENTING THE SELF

As I leaned into this parenting role with greater awareness, my understanding of child development—especially the subconscious mind—deepened. The electrical activity of the brain can be measured using an electroencephalograph (EEG), and what it shows us is profound: young children operate at much slower brainwave frequencies than adults.

For example, a two-year-old typically functions at about two cycles per second. This is equivalent to a frequency associated in adults with deep sleep or extremely drowsy states.

In these early years, the child's mind is essentially operating in a subconscious mode. The brain rapidly absorbs information without critical reasoning. This has massive implications.

The foundational programming that sets the tone for future beliefs and behaviours is built during a stage of life when the child lacks the intellectual framework to evaluate what they're receiving. Misinterpretation is common. Messaging is often incomplete or distorted. And yet these experiences become deeply ingrained, continuing to shape how we behave, think, and feel for years—often decades—afterwards.

For most of us, these original frameworks remain untouched and unchallenged. The stories we absorbed in childhood quietly accumulate weight and momentum, influencing everything from our relationships to our self-worth. Without conscious reflection and healing, the outcomes we experience as adults continue to mirror the shaky foundations laid in those early years.

Children, in their early stages, live from a beautifully egocentric worldview. They are the centre of their own universe, and everything that happens around them is interpreted through that lens.

Their subconscious programming is constantly being shaped by unfiltered external inputs. Repetition and emotion hardwire these messages into memory, creating the internal scripts that later become habits—some constructive, others limiting.

And while much of this learning comes from the environment, it's also shaped by each child's unique genetic blueprint. Their innate temperament, sensitivities, and strengths influence how they interpret the world and respond to it.

In this way, parenting isn't a one-size-fits-all process. I had to learn how to meet each of my children where they were, appreciating not only the messages I was sending but also how those messages were being received through their individual lens.

Parenting, then, is as much about self-awareness as it is about child-rearing. I must lead with love, compassion, and acceptance—not criticism or blame.

If I want them to listen, I must listen. If I want them to understand my perspective, I must be willing to understand theirs. It's not always easy. Being the role model they need involves confronting my own blind spots and limitations. It's a dance between knowing better and doing better, between reacting and responding.

Setting this example doesn't begin the moment a child is born—it begins with the work we do on ourselves beforehand. My emotional, physical, mental, and spiritual maturity determines my capacity to rise above egocentric reactions and consciously guide my children.

For both my husband and myself, the inner work was not optional. It was essential. Doing the work—individually and together—was necessary to become the kind of parents we aspired to be.

As Dr. Daniel Siegel reminds us, a parent's growth and emotional health profoundly shape a child's developing brain. "As parents become more aware and emotionally healthy, their children reap the rewards and move toward health as well."

If I want to raise children with resilience, confidence, and self-awareness, I must model that way of being. Parenting is not about perfect control, but about being a safe base from which children can explore life and make mistakes, and return to for love and guidance.

And as much as I guide them, they guide me. My children have been some of my greatest teachers.

Through them, I've uncovered hidden layers of my own story. I've re-examined how I was raised, what beliefs were passed down to me, and how I want to do things differently. The spiritual and physical influences of my own parents—already explored in earlier chapters—continue to ripple through my family line.

I want to honour those stories but also evolve them. Parenting has reminded me that we're not just raising children, we're rewriting legacies.

PARENTING THROUGH CONSCIOUSNESS

As wonderful as any family may be, there will always be moments when a child's perceived needs are not met. This can lead them to feel unseen, unheard, unloved, unworthy, misunderstood, not enough, or even too much. These emotional gaps, however small or unintentional, often leave subtle imprints. Some emotions get expressed outwardly, while others are held silently within.

Left unacknowledged, these internalised responses can evolve into survival-based emotions such as shame, guilt, insecurity, resentment,

THE BELIEF SHIFT

anger, or fear. And these emotions, in turn, may give rise to behaviours like avoidance, aggression, people-pleasing, withdrawal, or even physical symptoms of illness.

But what if these vulnerabilities didn't need to become burdens?

What if they could become gateways?

Practicing awareness of my emotional reactions has helped me understand not just what I feel—but why I feel it. I've learned that how I interpret a situation is less about what is actually happening, and more about what I believe it means about me.

Take this simple example: someone says, "You're doing that wrong." One person might interpret it as "I'm not good enough", and respond with defensiveness or shame. Another might hear the same words and think, "Oh, there's a better way? Tell me more", and respond with curiosity.

It's not the words themselves that matter most—but the beliefs we attach to them.

I wasn't always able to see it this way. My ability to interpret life with nuance and emotional clarity has grown over time, alongside my physical, mental, emotional, and spiritual maturity. As my self-awareness has expanded, so too has my ability to choose empowered responses, rather than default reactions.

This doesn't mean I always get it right—but it does mean I know how to pause and reflect.

What I think and feel shapes how I perceive myself and the world around me. And when I remember that I am the author of that inner story, I'm reminded that I can also edit it at any time.

In childhood, however, I didn't yet have this capacity. Back then, the interpretations I made were egocentric and emotionally immature. I often believed things happened because of me.

If something went wrong, my young mind would conclude, "I must have done something wrong", which quickly morphed into "I am wrong." This is not just my experience. Most children will make a similar assumption, thinking "It's my fault", which spirals out to beliefs like: "I am bad", "I am not worthy" or "I am not loveable". All, of course, are not true.

But beliefs easily become part of our identity. And when identity is formed through distorted conclusions, it often manifests in behaviour that reinforces the very belief we're trying to escape.

This is how a cycle begins: belief creates behaviour, which creates feedback that validates the belief. And round it goes. Identity, behaviour, and environment are deeply intertwined. When one is off-balance, the others are affected too.

Growing up, I often felt my dad wasn't around much. With a family of six to support and shift work to manage, I can only imagine the pressure he was under. When he was home, he was fixing things—cars, bikes, leaky taps—or trying to catch up on sleep.

Understandably, our noise often disrupted his rest. And when it did, we were met with a booming voice that sent us scattering. We knew that making noise meant getting into trouble (reconfirming the idea that we had "done something wrong").

Getting into trouble did not feel good.

From these moments, I unknowingly developed a belief system designed to keep me safe. Fear can do that. I learned that being loud was "bad", and therefore, I must be bad when I'm loud. So, the opposite must be true. I became quiet. I followed the rules. I stayed out of trouble.

I translated this into a new identity: being quiet and obedient means I'm good. My behaviour followed suit, and over time, this pattern became part of my personality.

Looking back, I can also see how my genetically adrenaline-sensitive nature—linked to my mesomorphic body type—played a part in how this response became imprinted. My version of being "good" was less about shrinking and more about holding a quiet form of defence to avoid judgment—almost like a subdued fight response wrapped in calm compliance.

Another person, with a different genetic makeup, might have responded to the same belief of "I am bad" with a more passive freeze, flight, or fawn response. On the outside, we might all look like "good girls", but on the inside, the motivations can be vastly different. The emotional consequence may instead come from a place of fear or disempowerment, rather than quiet resistance.

This is the subtle dance between nature and nurture, between genetic coding and lived experience. Together, they shape the personalities we come to identify with, often without us even realising how deeply rooted those patterns are.

But even years later, remnants of this belief still showed up.

My body would tense at raised voices. Arguments, especially among my sisters, would trigger a nervous system response. Even if the situation wasn't threatening, I felt a need to calm it down, to fix it, to protect everyone from the emotional discomfort.

These moments helped shape the "problem-solver" part of my identity. I became the helpful daughter, the tidy one, the good girl. I found safety and validation in order, responsibility, and achievement.

These traits brought praise, good grades, and trust from adults. But underneath them sat a younger part of me, trying to avoid trouble—trying to avoid the feeling of being seen as bad, of not being good enough.

Strength was born from that vulnerability. But so was a mask.

Every child, in some way, navigates this terrain—shaping beliefs from misunderstood moments and internalising meaning through the lens of a developing brain. Some beliefs empower us. Others limit us. Unless we become conscious of the stories we carry, we will unknowingly pass them on.

Awareness is the first step. Not just for healing ourselves, but for guiding our children.

Children are not born with the capacity to interpret the complexity of their emotional world. That's our role as parents—to develop ourselves so we can be the emotionally mature, safe presence they need.

Children need our regulation before they can regulate themselves. They need us to model what it looks like to be aware, to reflect, to pause, to own our part in things. And to rewrite our stories—so they can learn how to write theirs.

AWAKENING FROM THE SUBCONSCIOUS LOOP

Self-awareness involves becoming an astute observer of my life experiences and my reactions to them. The way I respond to comments or situations reveals key insights: not only about how far I've come in my personal development, but also where I still have work to do.

Through ongoing observation, I began noticing moments when I would abruptly shift into a defensive, negative state. A simple question from my husband—seemingly harmless—might provoke an unexpected, snappy reply. As he gently sought clarification, I would grow increasingly short-tempered, until a well-meaning conversation spiralled into a needless argument.

It took us both by surprise. This wasn't the outcome either of us wanted. It wasn't how I wanted to show up as a partner, or the behaviour I wished to model to our children. I loved him deeply, yet my reactions told a different story. I knew I could do better. He deserved better. I needed to explore what was truly driving these unwarranted reactions.

Upon deeper reflection, I recognised that my external behaviours were rooted in internal thought patterns and emotional responses—often operating beneath my conscious awareness. How I interpret a situation directly influences how I respond to it. But changing these ingrained interpretations required more than a surface-level fix.

I had attempted to act differently, to stay calm and respond with patience. And sometimes, it worked—until I was tired or distracted. Then, almost without warning, the old, defensive version of me would resurface.

To shift this dynamic, I had to go deeper. I needed to uncover the old programs—those subconscious patterns that may have once protected me but no longer served who I was becoming.

Behaviours, after all, are merely the tip of the iceberg. Beneath the surface lies a complex system: thoughts give rise to emotions, which in turn drive actions. And below thought itself is a foundation of deeply held beliefs—often inherited, ingrained, and unexamined.

To create lasting change, I had to rewire this foundation. I needed to write a new internal script, powered by conscious, empowered beliefs, that would override the inefficiencies of the old operating system.

It was time to build a new mind—one capable of generating fresh neural pathways and lasting transformation.

BELIEFS PASSED DOWN, BELIEFS RECLAIMED

During primary school, my sister and I would ride our bikes to school. One day on the way home, the chain on my bike snapped. I couldn't ride it, so I had to walk—an unexpectedly long journey.

Dad was a great help in teaching me how to service my bike. Over the years, it wasn't just the chain that needed fixing. He showed me how to repair punctured tyres and clean the spokes, derailleurs, and cables. A valuable lesson I learned that day, quite literally, was that a chain is only as strong as its weakest link. From then on, I always checked my bike before heading off and carried a spare tube, just in case.

What I didn't realise then is that we are only as strong as our weakest mental or emotional "link". There are many breaking points when forming new behaviours, but the biggest is the underlying belief we hold about ourselves. If I don't believe I'm capable of acting a certain way, I'm unlikely to even try. Beliefs are often more elusive than rusty chains or nails in tyres. So how do we uncover what's hidden?

Being prepared for likely problems is one strategy. It doesn't always expose root causes, but it equips us for challenges. With the bike, I didn't know the chain would snap, but I could have been more prepared, perhaps with a regular check or a small repair kit. These days, I always ride with spare parts. I don't want anything to go wrong, but I'm ready if it does.

When it comes to life's more important challenges, the equivalent of a bike check is awareness. Becoming an intentional observer of my behaviour allows me to notice patterns and ask better questions.

Take my husband's simple inquiries, for example. When I found myself reacting defensively, I started to dig deeper. I realised that it wasn't the questions that were the problem, but the meaning I attached to them: that I was being judged or doing something wrong. Somewhere along the way, I had formed a belief that being questioned meant I was inadequate. If I didn't believe that, there'd be no need to react with defence.

Awareness gives me the power to pause, reflect, and respond more consciously. It helps me ask myself: *"What's really going on beneath this reaction?"* Even if this belief was shaped by others, do I still want it to shape me?

Understanding the connection between beliefs and behaviours is crucial for shaping the life I want. When I take time to interpret what I observe, I can decide whether to keep a belief or update it.

Holding onto productive behaviours is wise since these usually lead to positive outcomes. It's the unproductive ones, the weak links, that hold me back. These are often driven by limiting beliefs, disempowering thoughts, and negative emotions.

For example, when I feel self-conscious at an event, I shrink instead of sharing my voice. I withhold my ideas and others miss out too. The ripple effect of a limiting belief reaches further than just me.

Most of us are held back not by one belief, but a cluster of interwoven ones. The good news is that changing one often loosens the grip of others. And usually, there's a dominant theme beneath them all.

For me, it was "not good enough". That belief coloured so many of my thoughts, feelings, and actions. Over time, with repetition and subtle reinforcement, this belief became ingrained. Once my brain was programmed, "autopilot" took over—and I wasn't even aware of it. I was living reactively, not intentionally.

Recognising this, I could see how my husband's questions triggered an old narrative. His words activated a story that was written long before we met. He was just a reflection of how I saw myself. My response had nothing to do with him and everything to do with the belief I'd internalised as a child. A belief formed by an immature, egocentric young brain trying to make sense of expectations, rules, and emotional responses.

Feeling the need to be perfect, to follow rules, not get in trouble, to be a "good girl"—these were the internal programs shaping my days. Anything that threatened that identity felt like judgment, triggering an automatic defence.

But awareness brings choice. I've begun to ask: *"Is this belief true? Is there another, more empowering one I'd rather hold? What belief feels authentic? Who do I want to be? How do I want to show up?"*

Facing these hidden parts of myself is uncomfortable. They've stayed buried for a reason. Sometimes I resist doing the work; other times I feel strong enough to go there.

In many ways, it feels like a rebirth—painful, yet filled with life-giving potential. There are new beliefs I can create, shaped not by old conditioning but by the wisdom of experience.

As I honour what feels true for me, I cultivate a space of unconditional love and acceptance for myself, and for my children, who are now weaving their own stories under my guidance.

RAISING AN AUTHENTIC FUTURE

Parenting is a journey filled with both challenges and triumphs. It is an exciting path where my past meets the present and helps shape the future. As I continue to navigate this terrain, I remind myself that while my children are deeply connected to my roots, they are also growing into their own unique identities.

Their world will look different from mine, and what worked for me may not serve them. Staying present and attentive allows me to honour their values and personalities while offering the guidance and perspective of my lived experience. As I continue to evolve, I can share my insights, love, and support in meaningful ways.

As Jane D. Hull wisely said, "At the end of the day, the most overwhelming key to a child's success is the positive involvement of parents."

In raising my children to be authentic, I strive to avoid blindly following societal expectations or outdated norms. Many of these externally driven values can lead to disconnection and disappointment when we mistake them as the path to happiness.

In the noise of parenting, alongside life's mounting pressures, it's easy to lose touch with ourselves. As explored earlier, identity extends beyond individuality; it encompasses the interconnected layers of our physical, emotional, mental, and spiritual worlds.

When I commit to living from my highest self, I naturally model a version of authenticity I hope my children can feel and embody—not just observe.

Reflecting on my own upbringing, I now better understand how deeply my parents influenced the shaping of my inner world. By illuminating subconscious beliefs that once held me captive, I've loosened their grip and reclaimed the power to choose how I respond.

With greater awareness, I'm able to act from intention, not instinct. I am committed to being the best mother I can be—but that means first being the best version of myself. It also means showing up fully for my husband, nurturing a partnership rooted in love, presence, and mutual respect.

Making space for joy and ease each day helps joy flow more freely through my life. My children are not only listening to what I say, but they are also watching what I do. They learn through my presence, my choices, and my energy.

That's why I focus on showing up as my truest self, as often as I can. There will always be challenges and unexpected turns, but if my husband and I remain grounded and united, we can continue to build the kind of relationships that matter most—to each other, and to our children.

To understand ourselves, we often have to look back—not to blame, but to see clearly. In tracing the threads of generational influence, we uncover not just the patterns we've inherited, but the possibilities we now hold.

Our families shape us in ways both seen and unseen. Their dreams, their fears, their coping strategies—they echo through our beliefs and behaviours. But we are not destined to repeat their stories. With awareness, we can choose which parts to honour, which to release, and which to rewrite.

This chapter has been a gentle unearthing of roles we've played, loyalties we've carried, and truths we're now reclaiming. It's not easy work. But it's powerful work. It brings us back to the roots so we can grow in a direction that feels authentic and free.

You do not have to carry it all. You get to choose what continues through you—and what ends with you.

Chapter Highlights

Destiny's Cradle:
The desire to nurture can surface long before motherhood, deeply rooted in childhood temperament and early life experiences.

Nurturing Their Dreams, Honouring Mine:
Life's detours often redirect us to greater alignment, even when they first appear as disruptions or disappointments.

The Reality of Parenthood:
Parental behaviours act as mirrors—children absorb more from what we do than what we say.

Parenting the Self:
Parenting invites us to become more self-aware.

Parenting Through Consciousness:
Understanding our emotional triggers helps break the cycle of reaction and fosters conscious parenting.

Awakening from the Subconscious Loop:
True transformation begins when we stop reacting on autopilot and start rewiring the beliefs beneath our behaviours.

Beliefs Passed Down, Beliefs Reclaimed:
Beliefs are the invisible scripts running beneath our behaviours—until we bring them to light, we continue to act from outdated programming.

Raising an Authentic Future:
Parenting is not about perfection but presence—modelling authenticity by showing up with intention, curiosity, and love each day.

REFLECTIVE QUESTIONS

1. When you reflect on your own childhood, what early signs of your temperament or passions can you now see more clearly?
   _____
   _____

2. Have you ever experienced a moment where life took an unexpected turn that ultimately aligned you more deeply with your purpose?
   _____
   _____

3. How did your own upbringing shape your expectations of family, love, and connection?
   _____
   _____

4. Do you see your childhood stories reflected in your current parenting style or relationship dynamics?
   _____
   _____

5. How do you respond to your child's emotional needs—and how does that relate to how your own were (or weren't) met?
   _____
   _____

6. What inherited beliefs have you consciously chosen to keep? Which ones are you working to release or rewrite?
   _____
   _____

7. What does authenticity look like for you right now—and how are you modelling that for your children?
   _____
   _____

Chapter 5

THE HEALING BEGINS

"Even the smallest shift in perspective can bring about the greatest healing."

JOSHUA KAI

Recognising the imprints passed down through generations offers us a powerful opportunity—not to carry them forward unchanged, but to consciously transform them. In understanding what we've inherited, we unlock the potential to heal not just for ourselves, but for those who came before us and those yet to come.

A powerful motivation for writing this book is to share my experience of self-healing—what's been possible for me and my family is also possible for you and yours. I am no different from you. If I can do it, you can too.

The healing that unfolded in our lives only reinforced the deeply supportive role we play as parents. The more attuned we are—to ourselves, our children, and the shifts that occur from day-to-day—the more consciously and compassionately we can respond. With this attunement, our responses become more aligned, and the outcomes more effective.

Healing rarely happens in isolation. When we experience transformation in one area of life, it naturally ripples into others. Change is possible. Healing is possible. And while it's ultimately a personal journey, it is never a solitary one. There are always unseen, yet powerful, connected energies guiding us—nudging us through the challenge and pointing us back to our strongest, most authentic self.

Children, in particular, rely on the presence and influence of the adults they trust. But we, too, can heal by leaning into trust—trusting ourselves, our intuition, and the higher frequencies of love and forgiveness that help us return home to who we truly are.

Throughout this chapter, I'll be sharing stories of my role as a parent and the influence I've had on my children's identities and growth. As you read, I encourage you to reflect on your own lived experiences. Where are you already shaping the dynamic within your family? Where do you hold the power to influence outcomes? Let these words serve as a gentle reminder of the profound imprint we leave on our children and the significant role we play in supporting their self-expression and self-healing.

Of course, healing will look different for everyone. There's no universal path, no perfect formula. What works beautifully for one person might fall flat for another. That's okay. Your job is not to follow a prescriptive plan but to explore and to discover the tools that resonate most with you and your family.

Choose to see self-healing as an act of radical self-compassion and true empowerment. No one outside of you can fully know what's best for you. When you take the reins of your own healing, you reclaim agency and with it, the freedom to create the wellbeing, peace, and joy you desire.

In the pages ahead, I'll share some of the tools and practices that have supported me and my family on our healing journey. My hope is that you'll see yourself as an active participant in your own life, with full permission to choose what feels right and let go of what doesn't.

BECOMING YOUR BEST HEALER

Healing is a conscious process—one that often begins with a mindful shift in beliefs, emotions, and habits. For me, it's been a dynamic interplay between mind and body, supported by a connection to a universal energy that gently holds them together.

There was a time when I lived much of my life on autopilot—unaware of many of my thoughts, feelings, and behaviours. Unsurprisingly, change felt out of reach. I couldn't shift what I wasn't even aware of. A daily practice of checking in and bringing gentle awareness to what was going on inside me became the first step. Connecting with my inner world and recognising the subconscious childhood programming that shaped my behaviour—often designed to protect against pain—was essential in beginning to heal it.

As children, we all encounter moments of pain. It's part of growing up. As adults, we're not exempt either. While uncomfortable, pain is not our enemy—it's feedback. It signals that we've interpreted an experience, either consciously or subconsciously, as fearful or unloving. This pain may be physical, emotional, mental, spiritual—or a layered combination. When we ignore it, that inner dissonance often manifests as a sense of powerlessness that cuts us off from our divine nature, leaving us feeling wounded and disconnected.

When I'm engulfed by powerlessness, it affects not only my emotions but also my beliefs and behaviours. I start to doubt my intuition. I no longer see challenges as opportunities. It's tempting, in those moments, to search outside myself for a quick fix—something or someone to distract me from the discomfort. At other times, I might suppress or deny my feelings altogether, hoping they'll go away if I just ignore them long enough. But as Carl Jung reminds us, "what you resist persists".

Pain cannot be released if I'm forcing it into silence. That tension only intensifies the pain, which will continue until it receives what it truly needs: presence, curiosity, and compassion. Think of a small child tugging at your sleeve, desperate for attention. If we turn and offer warmth and acknowledgment, they feel seen and soothed—and can happily move on. If ignored, they'll either escalate or withdraw, both of which lead to more challenging behaviour down the track. The same principle applies to our inner world. If we overlook the vulnerable parts of ourselves, we miss the opportunity to investigate what they're asking for and to respond with empowered action.

My years as a nurse gave me a front-row seat to many healing journeys. I helped patients integrate medical treatments into their lives and observed the powerful difference that personal engagement made. In my early career, most of my work was with adults. While some cases involved unavoidable accidents or inherited disease, many hospital admissions were rooted in chronic, preventable conditions—often the result of long-standing lifestyle choices. I saw again and again: when the body receives what it needs—at the right time, in the right way—it has a remarkable ability to heal. But that requires personal responsibility and intentional self-care.

When working with babies, the situation was different. They were completely dependent on the adults around them. Their healing relied on a network of caregivers—parents, medical staff, and allied health professionals. A healthy, present parent greatly increases the likelihood of a healthy child. In these cases, healing wasn't just about medicine—it was about connection, environment, and energy.

No matter the age, people in pain are vulnerable. They need support—but support alone isn't enough. True healing only occurs when we allow change. We can't stay the same and expect our lives, relationships, or health to magically transform. Healing asks us to step into a more empowered version of ourselves. To *see* the possibility of a healthy, whole self. To believe it's available. And to recognise that the world around us is always reflecting what lives within us.

Transformation begins inside. It comes from a place of courage, honesty, and willingness. But it's not something we have to do alone. We're supported—by people, by love, by life itself.

HEALING FROM THE INSIDE OUT

Over the past 15 years as a personal trainer, I've worked with many clients who wanted to change something about their lives—most often, their physical body. Many shared that they were stuck in "bad habits". They longed for transformation but struggled to build the new habits that would support lasting change.

They'd often say things like, "I know what to do—I just don't know how to do it consistently." They weren't lacking knowledge; they were looking for accountability and support to help them implement the actions they believed they "should" be taking—but deep down felt powerless to do.

While most of my clients were committed and showed up to our sessions consistently, many found it difficult to follow through when they were on their own. Week after week, some returned describing the same challenges that had initially brought them to me. Despite our work together, the routines of daily life—outside the gym—often pulled them back into old patterns. This left them feeling frustrated, disappointed, and defeated. "Why does this keep happening?", they would ask.

What I've come to realise—both in my clients and in myself—is that lasting change doesn't come from a single burst of motivation or an occasional session. It comes from a daily commitment to doing "the work". It's not really about willpower. Willpower often relies on force, and force eventually runs out.

What we need instead is *want power*—a connection to a deeper desire that pulls us forward. This desire becomes our internal motivator, helping us move through the resistance that so often shows up when we try to change. That resistance is usually fear in disguise—fear of discomfort, fear of failure, fear of letting go of who we've been.

And this is where the belief shift provides the magic. When we truly *want* something, and believe it's possible, we're more willing to meet that fear with compassion and move through it.

Going to the gym once a week won't create transformation if you still see yourself as someone who's unfit or struggling. Sustainable change comes when your identity shifts to, *"I am someone who values my health"*, or *"I am strong"*, or simply, *"This is who I am, so this is what I do"*. Our behaviours align with the beliefs we hold about ourselves. And when we change the internal story, our actions begin to reflect it.

Many people search for quick fixes—both in and out of the gym. Pills and prescriptions are often used to mask symptoms or manage conditions. While medications certainly have their place, there are countless lifestyle interventions that can create powerful results—without the side effects. But these require time, effort, and personal investment. And yet, the rewards are deeper and more lasting.

I tell my clients that the challenges we face in the gym are often metaphors for those we face in life. We can choose to lean into discomfort in pursuit of growth and strength—or stay within the bounds of what feels safe and familiar. Either way, our response to challenge is rarely limited to one area of life.

How we face difficulty is shaped by our early experiences—by the conditioning and beliefs we developed as children. If I want to heal, whether physically, emotionally, mentally, or spiritually, I need to change who I believe I am. I need to look inward and truly see myself. The outdated version of me—the one that no longer serves—

must begin to dissolve, so that a wiser, stronger version can take its place.

That means choosing to feel discomfort instead of fleeing from it. It means no longer seeing myself as weak or powerless. Instead, I must learn to meet my pain with compassion, to understand what it's asking of me. To really see it. By walking through the darkness, I can bring my pain into the light, where it can finally be transformed.

Until then, pain will continue to distract me—just like the small child tugging at my sleeve. But when I choose to acknowledge, validate, and embrace it, I build resilience. And with each act of self-compassion, I grow stronger and more able to face the challenges that once held me back.

PAIN, THE UNEXPECTED TEACHER

Several years ago, we were celebrating my father-in-law's 70th birthday. As part of our usual family tradition, we gathered at my husband's parents' home in a leafy suburb not far from where we lived. Friday nights were often lively with his five siblings, their partners, nieces and nephews—all coming together over shared food and conversation. But this particular Friday was different. A milestone birthday meant more people, more food, and even more celebration.

As a special gift, we brought a large blank canvas and vibrant blue paint with the idea of creating a communal piece of art. Each guest would leave their handprint on the 120cm-by-120cm canvas as a lasting memory of the day. My father-in-law loved the idea, and everyone joined in enthusiastically.

It was during this light-hearted moment that I noticed something troubling. My youngest son was struggling to press his hand onto the canvas. His expression revealed pain—not a typical reaction to an activity like this. He was ten years old: active, healthy, flexible. He'd been dancing for years, played basketball on weekends, swam regularly. This wasn't normal. I felt a rising concern. Something wasn't right. As the party carried on, a quiet worry began to take hold in me.

In the weeks that followed, our lives began to shift. We found ourselves moving between doctors' appointments, physiotherapy sessions, blood tests, X-rays, and bone scans. Eventually, we were given a diagnosis: Polyarticular Juvenile Idiopathic Arthritis—or JIA.

Polyarticular means five or more joints are affected. *Juvenile* refers to children under 16. *Idiopathic* means the cause is unknown. And *Arthritis*, in this case, meant pain, inflammation, stiffness, swelling, and warmth around multiple joints. In simple terms, my son had active arthritis in many areas of his young body.

As a nurse, I was familiar with what lay ahead—hospital visits, referrals, medications, and all the uncertainty that comes with a chronic diagnosis. While I understood these interventions were necessary, I also felt a deep internal pull toward hope and the need to stay grounded and positive for our family. We were told that long-term medication would likely be required and that a "cure" was not guaranteed.

The news was shocking. Arthritis is something most people associate with old age—not children. Like any diagnosis, it came with a flood of questions. How had this happened? How long had it been going on? Were there signs I had missed?

As I tried to process everything, I found myself revisiting earlier moments, wondering if I'd overlooked subtle clues. I recalled a period about two months earlier when my son had been unusually tired. One afternoon, he came home from school, went straight to bed, and slept until dinner—a rare occurrence. While both our boys had been very robust and healthy growing up, he did seem to carry a constant low-grade fatigue after that time and had begun withdrawing from his usual swimming and basketball sessions. We encouraged him to keep going, believing that staying active and social was best for his health. In hindsight, it may have caused more harm than good.

Naturally, the "mum guilt" crept in. Coupled with my identity as a nurse, I couldn't help but feel like I should have noticed sooner. Had life become too busy for me to recognise what was happening in my own child's body?

We followed the medical guidance as best we could. Despite that, his condition worsened. Three months after his diagnosis, he was admitted to hospital for steroid joint injections under sedation. It was just before Christmas. There was a growing anxiety in our family as the procedure approached. Thankfully, I was able to be with him during the sedation—holding his hand, calming his nerves, and sharing a few giggles as the sedatives took effect. Even in that moment, his playful spirit showed through. Maybe we were all getting a dose of the happy gas.

The weeks that followed were filled with regular appointments with his paediatric rheumatologist—at first every four weeks, then six, then eight. We waited and hoped. But I couldn't help thinking: *"What else could we be doing?"* Surely there were other strategies, other paths to support his body and spirit.

As someone who believes in the value of a holistic approach, I began to explore complementary therapies. We found a compassionate Chinese medicine practitioner, and my son began taking herbal formulas each morning. I was amazed by his willingness to drink them, despite the strong and generally unpleasant taste. We also added weekly acupuncture sessions and visits to a naturopath and kinesiologist.

Bit by bit, we noticed changes. Positive outcomes began to emerge. I genuinely believe these therapies helped support his healing, working alongside the conventional medical approach—not instead of it. They offered a more complete form of care, one that acknowledged the whole person, not just the illness.

LIVING WITH JIA: A LESSON IN RESILIENCE

Anyone who has managed life with a physical obstacle understands the challenges that come with reduced freedom. There can be strong resistance to situations that prevent us from fully experiencing life in the present moment. How we interpret and respond to these situations significantly shapes our experience. What one person may see as victimhood, another may embrace as victory—it all comes down to attitude and mindset. For instance, a cancer diagnosis can feel like a death sentence to some, or an opportunity for a life overhaul to others. As discussed in earlier chapters, much of our perspective is shaped by subconscious programming absorbed in childhood. We learn to see difficult life experiences as either setbacks or setups.

Living with Juvenile Idiopathic Arthritis was challenging, not only for our son, but also for his friends and family. School, sports, parties, and play can lose their joy when mobility is compromised, and painful flare-ups interfere. No two experiences are the same. The intensity of discomfort and which joints are affected can fluctuate by the hour, depending on the severity of JIA. Sometimes things were manageable; other times he needed extra help with everyday tasks like getting ready for school. Responses to illness vary widely among individuals—pain is never solely physical.

The psychological impact of chronic pain is well documented, often manifesting as depression, mood swings, anxiety, altered perceptions, and changes in cognition. How we perceive stress affects our bodies physically and chemically. Stress hormones trigger changes in brain chemistry that ripple far beyond the pain itself, influencing social, environmental, and personal adaptation.

At the peak of my son's symptoms, his school group went on a three-day interstate trip. Naturally, we worried about how he would cope without us. Thankfully, the teachers managed his condition with great care. But one day, the principal called me—and my heart sank. What had happened? Was he okay? How could I get there fast? What would she say?

The students had spent the day touring the Australian Institute of Sport, involving lots of walking and standing. As the pain escalated, my son struggled to keep up and began lagging behind. A teacher asked if a wheelchair was available. He refused, saying, "I'm fine. I don't need that. I'm not a cripple." But eventually, stubbornness gave way to acceptance, and he agreed to sit.

Over the phone, my mind raced to the worst. How much pain was he in? Was I a bad mother for letting him go? These unanswerable questions haunt parents. We were reassured everything was fine, and the wheelchair helped. His friends took turns wheeling him around, ensuring he felt included. I had to trust that he had the inner strength and support to be okay.

JIA affected his self-esteem and confidence. His sense of adventure, motivation to try new things, feelings of belonging, dance expression, and athleticism all suffered. Dancing, his passion since age three—twirling in the kitchen behind me while making lunch, or throughout the house—was put on hold. Something precious was missing.

Shifting focus from what he couldn't do to what he could do was key to building resilience. We read inspiring story books, made physiotherapy fun, and reminded him that this was just a temporary bump in the road. We assured him he would come through stronger and wiser. Dwelling on causes or uncertain futures distracted us from the present. Past experiences inform and sometimes predict our reactions—but observing the present moment and responding (not reacting) to what was truly happening was essential.

LISTENING TO THE QUIET WHISPER

While things had stabilised for my son both physically and emotionally, I couldn't shake the soft stirrings of a quiet inner voice. Something kept tugging at my awareness—a sense that we hadn't yet fully addressed the emotional component of his healing. One morning during meditation, I focused with more intention than usual. I asked clearly for guidance on how best to support my son's emotional healing. With gratitude in my heart, I released the request to the universe.

Later that same day, I came across an advertisement for a *spinal energy flow workshop* being held that evening, not far from where we lived. Was this the answer I had asked for? I took it as a sign and booked my seat.

A few hours later, I sat in a circle of curious adults, listening intently as the practitioner explained how energy moves through the body—and what happens when it doesn't. As she spoke, something clicked. Her words about energy blocks and the importance of flow switched on a light bulb in my mind. I felt I had uncovered something important, something that could help my son heal in a way that addressed more than just the physical symptoms.

Before I share what unfolded next, some background may be helpful.

Juvenile Idiopathic Arthritis (JIA), like many autoimmune conditions, remains something of a medical mystery. The immune system, designed to protect us, becomes confused and begins to attack healthy tissue—in this case, the joints—causing inflammation, swelling, and pain. The exact cause of JIA is unknown. It isn't inherited in a direct way, though genetic factors may play a role. And while lifestyle and environmental triggers are considered, no single explanation fits every case. What is clear is that JIA is nobody's fault.

Back at home, the light bulb was still glowing. From my science background, I understood that everything is made up of energy, including our bodies. For our systems to function optimally, energy must flow freely and smoothly. Any block or disruption can create pressure—much like a kink in a hose connected to a running tap. Even if water is available, it can't pass through the hose until the kink is released.

Our bodies consist of multiple systems—skeletal, muscular, nervous, endocrine, cardiovascular, lymphatic, respiratory, digestive, urinary, and reproductive. These systems don't just operate on a physical level—they are influenced by our emotional, mental, and spiritual states as well. Energy powers them all. In Eastern traditions, energy flows through the body via centres known as chakras—spinning wheels of energy that affect our health, mood, and behaviour. When these energy centres are blocked or misaligned, imbalances can show up in various areas of our life and health, often making it difficult to trace things back to a single cause.

As I sat in that workshop, the practitioner mentioned something that stopped me in my tracks: "an energy block at the level of the throat can present as arthritis".

Immediately, I thought back to an incident when my son was two years old. Most mornings, I went to the gym while the boys enjoyed playtime at the childcare centre. One hot morning, my youngest son experienced a frightening moment where his throat became restricted, and he couldn't breathe. It passed quickly, but at the time, it felt like forever. Physically, he recovered quickly. But what if, energetically, the experience left a residue?

Could that traumatic moment have created a blockage in his throat chakra, the energy centre associated with communication, expression, and flow? Like the kink in the hose, had that blockage quietly built up over the years—eventually manifesting as heat, pressure, and pain in his little joints?

The analogy of the hose came back again: the tap was on, the system was trying to function, but something was in the way. I began to wonder: *"What if all we needed to do was release that block?"* Could restoring energy flow help his body return to balance? How would we do that? Would it be easy? Would it work? Would the effects be immediate—or take time?

A flood of questions followed, as did a wave of doubt. Was I really considering energy healing? Was this too far-fetched? But deep down, I knew there was truth in what I was feeling. I had nothing to lose. And perhaps, just perhaps, we were about to step into a whole new world of understanding—the world of energy, and the healing power it held.

TURNING CHALLENGE INTO OPPORTUNITY

It's important to understand that feeling pain—whether physical, mental, or emotional—is not a sign of weakness. Pain is the body's natural and intelligent response to difficulty. It speaks in the language of protection and preservation. Denying, suppressing, or ignoring pain doesn't make us strong; awareness does. When we become willing to face our challenges—whether from the past, present, or those we anticipate in the future—we open a door to healing. We create an opportunity to choose a new way forward.

The meanings we give our experiences determine whether we are propelled forward or held back. Even in the midst of pain, we have agency. We can't always control what happens to us, but we can choose how we respond. That response might expand us or contract us. Either way, there is no right or wrong—just a shift in direction or focus. We are not powerless. We have the ability to respond. We are response-able. We carry the capacity to choose, and that choice shapes who we become.

I had already made the choice to help my son heal. But that also meant confronting my own discomfort—my fear of seeing him in pain, my feelings of helplessness, and the guilt that stirred inside me. I realised I needed to heal too. If I was to be the steady, loving guide he needed, I had to do the inner work alongside him. I didn't know exactly how, but I trusted that walking through this challenge together could lead us toward a greater opportunity—one we hadn't yet imagined.

We didn't ask for Juvenile Idiopathic Arthritis, but perhaps there was something more within it—a hidden invitation. Maybe it had come not *to* us, but *for* us. We live in partnership *with* life as it moves *through* us. Experiences shape who we become, but it's the meanings we assign to them that create our beliefs, our feelings, and ultimately, our actions.

I often return to the serenity prayer:

"God, grant me the serenity to accept the things I cannot change, the courage to change the things I can, and the wisdom to know the difference."

As parents, we make choices on behalf of our children. I was ready to make ones that integrated everything I knew—about the physical body, the mind, and the spirit. My nursing and science background gave me insight into the body's structure and function. My psychology studies helped me appreciate the emotional and cognitive impact of life events. And my upbringing, especially the teachings from my mother, reminded me of the innate spiritual power within us. Now, all these pieces had to be viewed through a new lens: energy.

What alignment was missing? What was stuck? And how could we turn this challenge into a transformation?

The next day, following the spinal flow workshop, I gently asked my son a few open-ended questions. I wanted to understand what he was holding onto emotionally, and how we might nurture that pain with love and compassion. At first, he struggled to find the words. I continued to hold space, rephrasing the questions, offering patience, and letting him know there was no rush. Eventually, the words came.

With a sudden exclamation and a rush of tears, something inside him released. His body softened. The tension seemed to evaporate, as if the emotions locked inside had finally found their exit. He looked lighter, freer—unburdened.

The next day, we noticed something remarkable: his joints moved without restriction. The pain was gone. It was as if his body had remembered how to flow again.

That healing came from seeing, honouring, and embracing the pain—not trying to fix or bypass it, but giving it permission to be. His younger body had responded the only way it knew how at the time. But now, we had the awareness, space, and support to do something different. We brought the hurt into the light. We gave it what it had always needed: love, understanding, and room to move.

Healing happens in the heart. The heart chakra—the centre of love, compassion, and unity—acts as a bridge between the upper and lower chakras. It integrates thought and feeling, body and spirit. When the heart is open, energy flows again, and the entire system finds its rhythm.

In the months that followed, his arthritis medication was gradually weaned and eventually stopped altogether. There were no further injections. No pain management. No flare-ups. And now, almost a decade later, he remains symptom-free.

Throughout our children's childhood, and especially during challenging times, we've always tried to explore different perspectives. We ask: *"What might this experience be trying to teach us? What's the opportunity hidden within this challenge?"* Sometimes the answers are easy to find. Sometimes, we have to look harder. But there is always a blessing. Always a gift.

This experience didn't just heal his body—it helped shape who he is today. Strong, resilient, creative, and expressive. A few years ago, after one of his dance performances, he turned to me and said,

"Mum, I'm so glad we got through the arthritis I had as a child. I wouldn't know what I would have done if I wasn't able to ever dance again. It certainly made me stronger."

It was a profound moment of gratitude. Not just for the healing, but for everything the journey had taught us.

When we are willing to meet our pain with compassion and curiosity, we unlock the potential for deep transformation. Healing does not always follow a linear or predictable path, but it does begin with the willingness to see things differently and to explore the connection between mind, body, spirit, and energy.

My son's recovery reminded me that true healing happens from the inside out—and that we each hold within us a unique code for thriving. In the next chapter, we will explore how to decode and personalise your own path to vitality, because the more you understand about yourself, the more empowered you become to live fully, freely, and well.

Chapter Highlights

Becoming Your Best Healer:
Healing begins with self-awareness. By gently turning inward, we can uncover the hidden beliefs and suppressed emotions that shape our behaviours, and learn to respond to our pain with compassion, curiosity, and conscious action.

Healing from the Inside Out:
Lasting change begins with a shift in identity. When we align our actions with who we believe we are—and meet discomfort with compassion—we begin to heal and grow from the inside out.

Pain, the Unexpected Teacher:
Pain, while never welcomed, can be a powerful teacher—calling our attention to what we've missed, inviting us to pause, reflect, and expand our view of what true healing might require.

Living with JIA: A Lesson in Resilience:
Resilience is nurtured by shifting focus from limitations to possibilities and by responding mindfully to the present moment rather than reacting to past pain or future fears.

Listening to the Quiet Whisper:
When the body speaks through illness, sometimes the answers lie in places beyond the physical, requiring us to listen to the quiet whispers of energy, intuition, and unseen emotion.

Turning Challenge into Opportunity:
True healing requires more than just treating symptoms—it calls us to listen deeply, to feel courageously, and to transform pain into power by embracing it with love.

REFLECTIVE QUESTIONS

1. What emotion or pattern have you been avoiding that may be calling for your attention, compassion, and healing?
   _____
   _____

2. What belief about yourself might need to change in order for you to embody the version of you who is already healing?
   _____
   _____

3. Has there been a moment in your life when pain led you to discover something deeper about yourself or someone you love?
   _____
   _____

4. How can you shift your mindset to focus on what is possible in your current situation, rather than dwelling on past setbacks or future uncertainties?
   _____
   _____

5. Is there a situation in your life where physical symptoms may be pointing to a deeper emotional or energetic imbalance waiting to be acknowledged?
   _____
   _____

6. Where in your life have you experienced pain that, when acknowledged and embraced, could become a powerful teacher or turning point?
   _____
   _____

THE BELIEF SHIFT

Chapter 6

THE BLUEPRINT WITHIN

"It is not in the stars to hold our destiny but in ourselves."

WILLIAM SHAKESPEARE

As I've continued my quest for vitality, I've become intimately familiar with the core pillars of health and wellbeing. The commonly referenced "big three"—nutrition, movement, and mindset—are undeniably important. But this framework often leaves something out: *you*. Your uniqueness. Your internal wiring. Your blueprint.

Most advice assumes a one-size-fits-all path to wellness. Yet so many people still struggle—not because they lack discipline, but because they're following strategies that don't fit. The truth is, we are not built the same. We don't respond the same. We don't thrive the same.

It's no secret that the biggest killers in our society—cardiovascular disease, dementia, cancer—are heavily influenced by lifestyle. We know that how we eat, move, think, and connect matters. But knowledge alone doesn't create transformation. What does? Personalised insight. A sense of relevance. Tools that actually match your biology, your environment, your stage of life, your goals.

That's where this chapter begins.

True wellbeing isn't about following someone else's formula—it's about uncovering your own. Your genes, your habits, your lived experiences, your unique chemistry all hold information that can guide your choices with precision. This is the heart of epigenetics and lifestyle medicine: we're not locked into a fixed path. We can shape our outcomes.

I've seen this firsthand—in my son's journey with illness, and in my own transition through the middle years of womanhood. What works beautifully for one body can be completely ineffective—or even harmful—for another. That's not failure. That's individuality. And when we embrace it, we move from confusion to clarity. From force to flow.

This chapter is an invitation to step into the driver's seat of your own health. Not with perfection, but with presence. With curiosity. With the understanding that your body isn't broken—it's communicating.

And when we learn to listen, we uncover the blueprint that's been there all along.

AN IDEA THAT CHANGED EVERYTHING

When creating strategies for lasting, effective outcomes, I find it helpful to start with the end in mind. Working backward from a clear vision of what I want helps me craft a roadmap to get there. I often ask myself: *"What is the outcome I'm hoping for? What does success look like? And what do I need to do to achieve it?"* Clarity on what success means *to me* sets the goalposts in the right place. Without it, I risk aiming mindlessly at something that may not even matter.

Success is highly individual and deeply personal. The Oxford English Dictionary defines success as "the accomplishment of an aim or purpose". But what aims are we talking about? For some, success might mean financial security or career achievement. For others, it could be living with purpose, having deep relationships, maintaining good health, or simply finding joy in everyday moments. To me, success also means growth—moving from restriction and limitation toward expansion and freedom. When it's aligned with my values and contributes to peace of mind, that's success worth pursuing.

So, what's *your* idea of success?

Getting clear about your definition of success can be a powerful awakening. Does it mean being happy, respected, wealthy, healthy, attractive, or admired? Where did that definition come from? Is it a reflection of your true desires—or something you inherited from childhood, school, culture, or family? Is your definition fuelled by the voice of your heart or the expectations of your head?

As a child, my idea of success included getting good grades, following the rules, avoiding trouble, being kind, and helping others. Later, it expanded to include respectable employment, a loving partnership, and creating a family. These ideals, though well-meaning, were often conditional. Over time, I began to realise that many of them weren't entirely *mine*. They were shaped by my upbringing, observations of my parents, and cultural cues. Unmet expectations could trigger feelings of failure—even when those expectations didn't reflect my deeper truth.

Now, with the clarity that adulthood brings, I can see that while the past shaped me, it doesn't have to define me. I've learned that I don't need to keep playing out patterns that no longer serve me. Life happens *with* us. Life is a gift that we don't just receive, but in fact have a hand in creating ourselves. We are not only participants but co-creators of our experience.

Understanding my mesomorphic biology through the exciting lens of epigenetics helped me see how my nature and nurture shaped my definition of success. For example, I've always been naturally action-oriented—driven by testosterone and adrenaline. Early on, that made me competitive and achievement-focused. But now, with a broader view, I replace "compete" with "create". I feel most alive when I'm in motion, engaged, and making a difference. That's not a flaw—it's my nature.

I've come to realise how important it is to stay in dialogue with the partnership between myself and life—to reflect, ask questions, and stay connected to what matters. Questions like: *"What do I care about? What do I want? What does life want to express through me?"* These aren't always easy to answer. Sometimes, they challenge my old programming. But they're essential for growth. They keep me aligned with who I'm becoming, not just who I've been.

To navigate this path authentically, I need to be clear on my values. My values define what I believe is important. They guide my decisions and behaviours. They also help me feel a sense of worth—both in who I am and in what I contribute. When I live in alignment with my values, I feel empowered, grounded, and more like myself.

Some values rise to the surface more clearly than others. I've come to notice that the things I'm naturally drawn to—the activities I enjoy and excel at—often point to those deeper values. They're the moments when I feel most alive, fully present, and in flow. For me, that happens when I'm moving my body, lost in conversation, solving problems, or diving into something new about health and human potential.

When I reflect on those sparks of joy and presence, I notice recurring themes. I've always been energised by learning, especially about health and human potential. I've also always loved sharing what I learn—whether through coaching, writing, or in conversation with someone curious (and hopefully not trying to escape!). These clues tell me where my true interests lie and where I can make the biggest impact.

Movement is another essential thread in my blueprint. My body feels most alive when it's in motion. Whether I'm exercising, dancing, or simply moving through the day with purpose, physical activity brings me joy, vitality, and connection to myself. It's not just something I *like*—it's something I *need*. My body was built for it. It's wired into my DNA.

Expression—through movement, through words, through connection—is how I bring it all together. Writing, speaking, and coaching give me ways to channel what matters most: contributing, connecting, and inspiring change. These aren't random preferences. They're clues, encoded in me, pointing toward who I truly am and how I'm here to show up.

Interestingly, these very patterns were confirmed through my epigenetic assessment. Seeing my natural strengths and preferences reflected back to me was powerful and validating. It affirmed what I already knew at a deep level—and it helped me trust that I was on the right path.

"I love to learn and like to be well informed. I am energetic and full of ideas. I may contribute strongly to a profession that allows me to express myself freely. I enjoy communicating, guiding others, and persuading people. This might allow me to excel in sales, teaching workshops or training, or doing any job that allows me to relate to people…"

That's a snippet from my personal epigenetic profile. And it's remarkably accurate. It's me. That kind of insight reminds me why personalisation matters. When you know yourself—your biology, your values, your environment—you can make choices that align with the life you were meant to live.

UNLOCKING THE TREASURE WITHIN

Unlocking the lid to reveal the gold I carry within comes from looking at my life holistically—from every angle, with honesty and care. Understanding how nature and nurture intertwine helps me appreciate the importance of aligning my biology with my environment and lifestyle. When I nourish my biological needs through movement, meaningful expression, and social connection, I feel more grounded. This groundedness gives rise to a quieter inner world—one where I can hear the gentle whispers of my heart. But I need my body to be vibrant and healthy to receive those messages.

Living in alignment with my natural gifts—and accepting both my strengths and limitations as valid parts of me—removes any lingering shame or confusion. It brings clarity. I am who I am. It's written in my biology, and I can learn to live in harmony with it. Even more exciting, I've learned I can read this biology like a map—a guide to help me navigate life more authentically.

For me, optimising health became a more exciting and rewarding project once I discovered the world of epigenetic personalisation. With open awareness, I've been learning how to create a healthy flow between my inner and outer worlds. I now see many parallels between my internal makeup and the experiences I encounter in the external world. There's a deeper connection at play—a sense that everything is part of the same thread. That awareness helps me surrender more fully to life, trusting that a higher power is gently expressing itself through me. My greatest success comes from removing resistance to that natural flow.

Vibrant joy doesn't come from achieving a single milestone—it comes from exploring the many dimensions of what it means to be fully human. For me, that includes understanding how my personal values, my unique biology, and my lifestyle intersect and influence each other. When I align these parts of myself, I feel more whole. Taking physical and emotional action serves as a kind of inner compass, guiding me toward the life I'm meant to live—and allowing me to help others through the sharing of my gifts.

When I look back now, I see that I've always been reaching toward this kind of expression. Playing sports—both individually and in teams—allowed me to satisfy my internal drive for movement and leadership. It gave my energetic nature a place to land. As a child, I struggled with being still. I wanted to move. I wanted to express myself. I didn't always have the words, but I had the will. Sometimes, my need for expression showed up as conflict—especially when I felt that my values were being challenged. Whether spoken or unspoken, internal friction would build, and I'd feel compelled to act in ways that aligned things with what felt "right" to me.

There were also times I didn't have enough confidence or trust in myself to speak openly. I'd hold back. That internal pressure would build into quiet anger or hidden resentment. On the surface, I might appear cooperative—but underneath, I was wrestling with a disconnect between how I felt and what I could express. Now, I see those moments not as failures, but as clues. Each thought, feeling, and behaviour was a puzzle piece. With time and distance, I've gained the perspective to step back and see the full picture more clearly.

Owning this reality as part of my identity has helped me surrender with peace. It has also taught me that we are all *meant* to be different. Our differences aren't obstacles—they are contributions. Together, our uniqueness creates a powerful mosaic, greater than the sum of its parts. Like pieces of a jigsaw puzzle, we need our distinct edges to fit into the bigger picture. If all the pieces were the same, nothing would stand out—and nothing would connect.

SEEING THE WHOLE PICTURE

Learning about epigenetics—and how my environment and lifestyle influence my biology—has given me the opportunity to get more personal with my life experience. It's deepened my understanding of myself beyond nutrition, movement, and mindset, expanding into areas like sleep, light exposure, socialisation, and stress. To show up in the world as my best self, I need to feel energised, centred, and ready for whatever life brings. That readiness comes from aligning all parts of me—body, mind, heart, and spirit.

Fulfilling many different roles requires different skill sets, but they all stem from one important place: an inner confidence that comes from being anchored in who I truly am. When I live from this place—connected to my biology and aligned with my values—I feel the ease and flow that wellness brings. This self-awareness has been transformational not only for me, but also for my family.

One of the most practical and empowering shifts has been in how I move my body. I've always been an early riser and a morning exerciser. That hasn't changed—but now, I understand *why* that works for me. Morning light exposure and short, varied workouts support my biology. I've also learned to prioritise rest and recovery to avoid burnout and maintain my energy. For my biology, intensity must be balanced with sustainability. Recovery has now become my secret weapon.

But what works for me isn't right for everyone—and this is where personalisation shines. My eldest son, for example, has a "night owl" biology. Early morning workouts were draining and stressful for him. Once we adjusted his exercise routine to better match his natural rhythm—later in the day—his energy, mood, and muscle development noticeably improved. Now, while I'm rising with the sun, he's still fast asleep. And when I'm winding down at night, he's in full academic flow.

Our different needs and preferences have helped us give each other permission to honour what feels right—and stop trying to force each other into a one-size-fits-all mould.

This awareness has carried through to other areas too—like how we experience and interpret relationships. For me, social interaction is energising and positive. It's about joy in the moment and a chance for creative self-expression. For my eldest son, it's about forming deep emotional connections, unconditional support and generosity. Lots of alone time and trust of others are foundational to feeling safe in relationships for my youngest son. Recognising these differences allows us to operate from a place of acceptance rather than resistance.

We also differ in how we orient our internal focus. I tend to be present-oriented and self-driven, which can feel exciting but also make me more sensitive to external feedback. Phrases like "You're too much", "You're too loud", or "You're too opinionated" used to trigger an inner conflict. I'd wonder whether I needed to tone myself down to be accepted. But now, I understand this is just part of my natural design—my energetic wiring—and that awareness softens my response. Instead of defaulting to self-doubt, I can choose more supportive narratives: *"I am worthy as I am", "I am enough" or "I have valuable ideas to share".*

When we understand where our values, natural strengths and vulnerabilities lie, we can make more informed, empowered choices. Thinking, feeling, and acting in ways that align with our unique design allows us to move through life with more grace and authenticity. When we stop striving to become someone else and start honouring our own biology, life gets easier. We begin to see ourselves with greater compassion and clarity. This self-awareness becomes our foundation—not just for better health, but for a life of deeper joy, ease, and purpose.

True success isn't about striving to meet someone else's standard. It's about uncovering what feels *right* for *you*—and living it fully.

Your unique code isn't just something to know—it's something to *live*. When your daily habits and choices reflect your inner truth, life begins to flow with less resistance and more resonance. What once felt confusing starts to feel aligned.

As I continue walking this path, I realise my true self was never lost—just layered beneath years of expectation, conditioning, and distraction. And like any blueprint, it needed the right conditions to emerge: presence, patience, and a willingness to live with intention.

Now that we've uncovered the genetic, energetic, and emotional threads that shape who we are, the next step is integration. In the following chapter, we'll explore what it means to live in alignment—to embody this self-knowledge in the everyday, and to stay connected to what matters most.

Because when your outer world begins to reflect your inner truth, you don't just live—you *thrive*.

Chapter Highlights

An Idea that Changed Everything:
Defining your own version of success—based on your biology, values, and lived experience—allows you to live with greater alignment and purpose.

Unlocking the Treasure Within:
Living in sync with your natural gifts, biology, and environment is like unlocking a personal treasure map. When you express who you are without resistance, you experience more clarity, creativity, energy, and connection.

Seeing the Whole Picture:
Embracing your full story—biology, values, experiences, and emotions—brings clarity and compassion to your identity. Recognising your patterns and responses helps you understand who you are, what you need, and how you relate to the world.

REFLECTIVE QUESTIONS

1. Where in your life have you been following generalised advice that doesn't truly reflect your individual needs or preferences?

   _____
   _____
   _____

2. What beliefs about success have you inherited, and do they still feel true for you?

   _____
   _____
   _____

3. What are the environments, activities, or experiences where you feel most fully yourself—and how often do you allow yourself to be there?

   _____
   _____
   _____

4. What parts of your story—past behaviours, reactions, or tendencies—might make more sense when viewed through the lens of your natural wiring and values?

   _____
   _____
   _____

Chapter 7
STAYING TRUE

"In a world where you can be anything. be yourself."

ETTA TURNER

To stay true is to live in alignment with your authentic self, without hiding behind masks or armour. It doesn't mean having all the answers or becoming some perfected version of yourself. It means showing up as you are, moment by moment, with honesty and presence.

Staying true to yourself is less about striving, and more about remembering. Remembering what you value. Reclaiming your worth. Tapping into what feels nourishing. What makes you feel alive?

Alignment reveals itself in the quiet, often overlooked spaces—when your actions reflect your values, when your relationships sustain you rather than drain you, and when your choices are guided by clarity instead of conditioning.

To live this way isn't always easy. But it is deeply freeing. It invites a slower, more honest rhythm—one rooted not in performance, but in presence. This chapter explores what it means to return to that place of inner alignment, again and again, and to build a life that reflects who you truly are—not just on the inside, but in the world around you.

THE EVERYDAY MIRROR

Living within the flow and rhythm of a long relationship means there are days that feel uneventful and mundane, while other days are filled with joy and amazement. My husband and I have been lovingly married for over twenty years. We know each other's rhythms, quirks, and shadows. And still, there are days where I surprise myself—where the mirror he holds up to me reveals parts I didn't know I'd tucked away. Like the time I reacted sharply to a small comment he made about how I unloaded the dishwasher. My defensiveness caught me off guard. It wasn't about the plates—it was about being seen as careless. In that moment, I recognised an old wound around needing to prove my worth through doing things "right". His simple observation became an invitation to notice what still needed healing.

There's a special kind of intimacy that comes from being fully seen and still fully loved. It's beautiful. And terrifying. And ultimately liberating.

When we're honest, we realise that our closest relationships often reflect the parts of ourselves we've polished—and the parts we still hide. My husband has become a mirror I never asked for but deeply needed. Not because he corrects me, but because his presence invites me to witness myself with both tenderness and accountability.

This mirror isn't always gentle. It's real. Sometimes it shows the edges of my impatience, the scars of childhood roles, or the flicker of fear I thought I had healed. But it also reflects my growth, compassion, playfulness, and the deep well of love I have to give when I feel safe to be me.

Love—whether romantic, familial, or self-love—has the capacity to alchemise discomfort into wisdom. True alignment isn't about perfection; it's about integrity. It's the courage to live without pretence. To honour the wisdom of your body, heart, and intuition over external expectations. And it's in the quiet spaces of daily life— those unfiltered moments—that this alignment is tested and refined.

A FAMILY IN FLOW

Years ago, during a quiet beach holiday, our family began a tradition that continues to shape how we show up for each other. As the end of the year fast approached, we gathered around the dinner table with salt in our hair and sand still clinging to our feet. Someone (it may have been me) suggested we share our individual intentions for the new year ahead. It was a simple idea. But the ripple effect was profound.

One by one, each of us—my husband, our children, and I—spoke about how we wanted to feel, what we hoped to experience, or what we wanted to release. There were no rules. Just presence. Honesty. And curiosity.

That week unfolded differently. Conversations were richer. Laughter came easier. Frustrations were met with more grace.

Something sacred had been stirred—not by the words themselves, but by the act of listening and witnessing.

What we didn't realise then was that we were creating a container for alignment. A space where each of us could show up as ourselves and be met with acceptance. It became less about getting along and more about being real.

Since then, we've repeated this ritual in different ways—sometimes during holidays, other times around the dinner table after a hectic week. Each time, it reminds us that connection isn't built in grand gestures but in the willingness to be seen and heard. To be supported and to provide support.

When we live in alignment, it doesn't just affect us—it radiates. Our presence becomes an invitation. Our groundedness calms the nervous system of the room. Our authenticity gives others permission to exhale. We stop performing and start relating. That's how families thrive—not in perfection, but in flow.

SACRED SPACES OF CONNECTION

Long-term relationships are sanctuaries where the soul learns to stretch and soften. They're not always comfortable, but they can be profoundly healing.

There was a time early in our marriage when I confused harmony with silence. I avoided conflict at the expense of truth. I thought love meant keeping the peace, even if it meant swallowing my needs. But the cost was disconnection—from myself, and eventually, from him.

What I've learned is that sacred connection is built not on flawless communication, but on mutual respect and the courage to be emotionally honest. Sometimes it requires difficult conversations and uncomfortable emotions.

One of the greatest gifts we can offer our loved ones is a safe space to evolve. A space where they can shed old skins, revisit old wounds, and explore new edges—without fear of rejection. In return, we need that same spaciousness. That same grace.

It takes time and conscious effort to cultivate this kind of intimacy. It requires presence. Emotional literacy. And above all, trust. Trust that when we speak from the heart, even to expose the messy parts, love can hold us. Trust that truth, when shared with kindness, brings us closer—not further apart.

These sacred spaces don't always look dramatic or deep. Often, they're built in micro-moments: a hand on the back when we're tired, a willingness to listen when the other doesn't yet have the words, a glance that says, "I see you, even now."

True connection calls us into alignment—not by force, but by gentle invitation. It reminds us that authenticity isn't selfish. It's sacred.

THE ENERGY OF TRUTH

Truth feels different. Even when it's hard, it brings a quiet relief—an inner exhale. When we speak or live from that place, the body softens. The nervous system settles. We feel grounded, clear, and free.

In contrast, when we betray what we know deep down, something tightens. We hold our breath. We shrink. We resist. These moments are not signs of failure, but invitations to return to truth—to shift the story we're believing, and to realign with what we know in our bones.

Our energy doesn't lie. It always tells us when something isn't true for us. Listening to it is how we come home.

When we hide who we really are—even from the people we love—it creates an inner tension that's hard to name but easy to feel. It's an energetic contraction. A holding in. A dimming down. And over time, that internal pulling back starts to show up in our outer world: as resentment, disconnection, exhaustion, or even illness.

When we feel drained, contracted, or resistant, it's rarely because we're broken—it's often because we're believing something that isn't true. Alignment isn't forced—it's felt. And the body always knows. We may not always recognise it, but over time the body tells us—offering quiet signals for those willing to listen.

Early in my adult life, I became a master of subtle hiding. Smiling when I wanted to cry. Agreeing when I wanted to challenge. Appearing calm when I was storming inside. It wasn't conscious at first. It was adaptive. Survival dressed as politeness. A learned behaviour that seemed to serve me well.

But eventually, the cost of that misalignment caught up with me.

I began to notice patterns repeating—people and situations that mirrored back the very things I was afraid to face: my need to be heard, seen, known. I saw how easily my energy dropped when I ignored my inner knowing. And how something shifted—subtly but powerfully—the first time I chose truth over comfort. Not to harm, but to heal.

That was the beginning of a different kind of strength.

Living in alignment with ourselves requires courage—not the loud, dramatic kind, but the quiet, daily kind. The kind that speaks up when silence feels safer. That sets boundaries when people-pleasing would be easier. That allows truth to rise, even when our voice shakes.

It's not about bulldozing others with our beliefs or declaring ourselves "right". It's about honouring what's true for us—while also respecting what's true for them. It's about finding the brave middle ground where honesty and compassion can coexist.

Courage, like any muscle, grows with practice. Every time we choose presence over performance, truth over protection, self-respect over self-abandonment—we reclaim a little more of ourselves. And with that reclamation comes freedom.

There is quiet power in saying, *"This is who I am. I may not have it all figured out. But I'm here, and I'm willing to show up—fully."*

That's not a weakness. That's the beginning of realignment. And realignment is where transformation begins.

ORDINARY TO BRILLIANT

As a child, I remember watching my mother cook the evening meal while I worked through my homework at the dining table.

She'd softly hum along to the tune on the radio, one hand stirring a simmering pot, the other reaching for ingredients without missing a beat. Simple food, prepared with quiet care. I didn't realise it then, but I was witnessing something sacred: the harmony of attention, love, and purpose woven into an everyday act. That was alignment—not in a flashy or obvious way, but in how fully present she was. No rushing. No resentment. Just a kind of peace that shaped the whole atmosphere around her.

We tend to overlook these moments, yet they are often where the most profound shifts occur. When we meet the ordinary with care, we return to ourselves. Alignment doesn't always come from certainty or grand transformation—it comes from the willingness to be fully present, even in the mess, even in the mundane.

But presence isn't always easy. Life offers friction on purpose. Growth needs resistance. Without it, we'd never develop the strength to discern what truly matters. The challenge is not to avoid resistance, but to engage with it as a mirror, a teacher, a guide.

I remember a moment recently when I snapped at my husband for something as small as leaving the laundry on the floor. It wasn't really about the laundry. The irritation came from deeper down—from the pressure of feeling unseen and overstretched. That flash of anger revealed something I hadn't paused to acknowledge: a longing to be supported, not just helped. Resistance isn't wrong—it's revealing. It shows us where something inside is asking for attention, where an old belief or unmet need may no longer fit the truth of who we've become.

When we meet resistance with compassion rather than judgment, we open the door to brilliance. Not a polished or perfect brilliance, but one born of presence, truth, and growth.

Some of my most aligned moments have come not from clarity, but from confusion. Not from smooth paths, but from the stumbles. The tension of not knowing invites a deeper knowing. It asks us to trust something within.

Alignment is not something you chase. It's something you allow. A natural buoyancy returns when we're no longer weighed down by expectations or old identities. The more we release, the more easily we rise. And sometimes, the most brilliant shifts come quietly—in the middle of an ordinary day.

LIVING A REAL LIFE

There's a subtle war many of us fight—a war between who we are and who we think we need to be. We strive, compare, and contort. We chase approval, wear masks, and deny desires that don't fit the image.

But living in alignment means coming home to yourself, again and again.

For much of my life, I carried the weight of perfectionism. It was inherited, praised, and rewarded. But it was also exhausting. It kept me on edge—hyper-vigilant, always measuring, never quite arriving.

What I've come to understand is that alignment is not about getting it right. It's about recognising when something feels wrong. It's about learning the language of your body and energy and using that information to return to truth.

If something feels heavy, constricting, or depleting—it's likely not in alignment. That's not a reason for shame. It's a signal. A doorway.

We now know through epigenetics that we are not hardwired to repeat our past or our parents' pain. We can turn genes on and off through lifestyle, environment, belief, and emotion. In the same way, we can rewire patterns of self-abandonment—by making one conscious choice at a time.

Each day is an opportunity to notice: Am I contracting or expanding? Am I in truth or in defence? Am I choosing from fear or from freedom?

Every moment is an invitation to return to yourself.

To pause when your heart clenches.
To breathe before saying yes.
To listen to the whisper beneath the noise.

To soften instead of striving.
To ask: "Is this true for me?"

Staying true to yourself isn't a one-time decision. It's a daily practice. A tender, sacred rebellion in a world that profits from our disconnection.

And yet, when we align, we begin to lead from within. We create lives that feel good on the inside, not just look good on the outside. We become steady in uncertainty, kind in conflict, and anchored in love.

That's the gift of alignment. Not that life becomes easier, but that we meet it as our whole selves—real, radiant, and rooted in truth. A truth that is founded on the belief that we are already abundant, we are already full of love. We are love.

BELIEVE THE LOVE YOU ARE

I believe that our natural state is love. Brilliance. Wholeness. But life teaches us otherwise. We internalise fears, absorb conditioning, and forget our original essence.

When I am aligned with love, I feel weightless. Clear. Alive. That's when I know I'm home. But when I slip into striving, controlling, proving—I feel resistance. My energy tightens. That too is a signal, not of failure, but of misalignment. A belief asking to be seen and softened.

I used to think boundaries were about control. That strength meant performing resilience. But now I see that true power is gentle. It's saying no with love. It's saying yes without guilt. It's resting when the world tells you to grind. It's knowing you are enough—without needing to earn it.

Fear wears many masks: ambition, discipline, self-help. It says, *"Become more and then you'll be worthy."* But love says, *"You already are."*

Each emotion we feel is a guide. Sadness, anger, anxiety—they are not signs that we are broken. They are messengers, pointing us to a place within that longs for attention, truth, or release.

The more I pause to feel, the more I notice: energy always tells the truth. Beliefs become visible in the body before they rise to the mind. If I feel depleted, it's often because I've picked up a story that isn't mine. Or stayed too long in one that is no longer true.

That's why staying true to ourselves is not a one-time awakening—it's a daily choosing. To return. To soften. To shift from fear to love. To notice when we've resisted what is and gently realign.

You don't need to be fixed. You need to be remembered. Realigned. Loved back into the wholeness you've always been.

And when you live from that place, the world around you begins to shift—not because you're trying to change it, but because your energy invites something deeper to emerge. You become a lighthouse. A reminder. A radiant presence in a world that so often forgets its own light.

What I tell myself becomes my truth. So I choose wisely. I choose joy. I choose love. I choose the beliefs that serve my highest good.

As I've learned to live in greater alignment—with my truth, my body, my relationships, and my inner rhythm—I've come to see that this personal alignment naturally spills outward. It opens the door to something larger than myself. Because when we live in integrity with who we are, we begin to ask different questions—not just *"Who am I?"* but *"Why am I here?"*

Alignment to who we are becomes the fertile ground from which a deeper sense of meaning can grow. And so we step forward, heart open, into the greater invitation: a life shaped not only by authenticity but by purpose.

Chapter Highlights

The Everyday Mirror:
Close relationships act as mirrors, revealing both our growth and our shadows.

A Family in Flow:
Living in alignment influences not just the self, but family dynamics and emotional tone.

Sacred Spaces of Connection:
True intimacy is built on emotional safety, mutual respect, and honest communication. Sacred connection arises when we allow each other room to evolve.

The Energy of Truth:
Our energy state is an accurate signal of when we are living in alignment—or not.

Ordinary to Brilliant:
Resistance and confusion are not barriers but pathways to growth and inner brilliance.

Living a Real Life:
Perfectionism disconnects us. Returning to presence and inner truth restores alignment.

Believe the Love You Are:
Our natural state is love. Emotional patterns reveal hidden beliefs that shape our lives.

REFLECTIVE QUESTIONS

1. In what ways has a long-term relationship reflected truths about yourself?
   _____
   _____

2. What small gesture could bring more intentional presence to your relationships?
   _____
   _____

3. Where in your life do you feel a subtle energetic contraction—and what truth might be buried there?
   _____
   _____

4. What does courageous communication look like for you in this season of life?
   _____
   _____

5. How do you respond when something feels "off"—and what would it look like to listen more deeply to that signal?
   _____
   _____

6. What belief about yourself are you ready to shift—and what new story are you willing to live?
   _____
   _____

7. What does it mean for you to live in alignment with love today—in one small but meaningful way?
   _____
   _____

THE BELIEF SHIFT

Chapter 8

A BIGGER PURPOSE

"The privilege of a lifetime is to become who you truly are."

CARL JUNG

Unravelling the mystery of why I'm here has become a quiet, ongoing conversation within me. Perhaps it's not a mystery at all. Maybe purpose isn't something hidden to be found, but something simple and sacred—something that reveals itself in the ordinary rhythms of daily life. Whether you believe your reason for being is to complete your to-do list or you feel called toward something larger, one truth seems universal: we're all seeking meaning.

As I move through my fifth decade—and as life moves through me—I find myself less interested in chasing purpose and more interested in allowing it. For years, I searched outside myself, driven by a desire to *be more*, *do more*, *know more*. But slowly, that striving softened into something more spacious. I began to see that what I'd been chasing wasn't out there—it was already within me. Purpose, I've come to believe, is not something to achieve. It's something to remember. Something to become.

And becoming takes presence.

True purpose doesn't arrive through force—it rises through connection. It's not just about what I'm here to do, but who I'm here to be. A frequency I tune into, not a role I perform. When I am still, when I listen, I feel it: a quiet pulse of meaning guiding my choices from within. For me, that pulse feels like love moving through me. Like spirit. Like life itself.

This chapter is about that kind of purpose—the kind that isn't dictated by titles, roles, or accolades, but by alignment. A living rhythm between your soul and your everyday life.

But to live this way, we have to explore some deeper territory:

- What is desire, really? Could it be a form of divine direction—a spiritual GPS?

- What happens when we stop resisting life and allow it to move through us?

- What if our greatest power lies not in the striving, but in the surrender?

We'll explore these questions through the lens of presence**,** alignment, and the alchemy of desire. We'll look at how the energy behind our longing can lead us back to our truest self—not by pushing harder, but by softening into trust.

As I write this, I feel vulnerable. Purpose is tender terrain. We each hold our own meaning. Some of us have been searching for decades; others might just now be feeling the stir. But if you've made it this far in this book, I trust you're ready to explore what purpose means for *you*—not just as a concept, but as a living presence in your life.

My hope is that this chapter gives you permission to loosen the grip on who you think you should be—and to feel the quiet, powerful presence of who you already are.

LIFE IS THE PRESENT

Often, we are so busy with all our activities and commitments that we barely take a moment to stop, reflect and be grateful for all we have. Life is a gift to be appreciated and enjoyed, but many of us fail to recognise the present that it is. In fact, it almost seems like a badge of honour to be busy. Listen to how people reply when you ask how they are. Count the times you hear, "Oh I am so busy!" or "Life is incredibly busy!" or "I'm flat out, run off my feet!" Being busy has become a signal of importance—or sometimes a cry for help.

I've certainly fallen into the busy-ness trap myself. At times, I wonder whether I create that state unconsciously, filling the space instead of facing the stillness.

Over the past few years, I've made a conscious effort to slow down. I've been training my body and mind to focus on what's within rather than what's outside. Letting go of the pressure to achieve and the expectations of all the "shoulds" has been liberating. Practices like meditation, yoga, walking, and time in nature bring me back to myself. They help me experience presence—physically, emotionally, spiritually. They help me remember who I am.

One of the most powerful tools I've discovered is the breath. When I bring my awareness to it, my breath becomes an anchor in the present moment. I inhale what I need. I exhale what no longer serves me. Each breath reminds me that I can let go with ease. I don't need to force, control, or strive—life moves through me effortlessly when I allow it.

I'm reminded of a beautiful Buddhist teaching: "I wholeheartedly welcome whatever arises, having given up the idea that things should be other than what they are." The breath, like life itself, doesn't need our control. It knows what to do. It simply flows—effortlessly, wisely, faithfully.

Each breath is a sacred exchange. A giving and receiving. A balancing of energy. It is a force that animates our human form—an unseen, yet deeply felt, current of love. Though invisible, it is no less real. Just as we feel heat from the sun or music in the air, we can feel this spiritual energy too—especially when we breathe with intention.

When I sense tension in my body, I imagine breathing into an open heart. I visualise expansion—like a balloon filling with love-fuelled energy, softening any places of contraction. Sometimes I picture colour moving in and out, dissolving what's been stored and healing what's been hidden.

This is how I return to presence.

Living in the present moment, with presence, is a powerful act of purpose. I've tried filling the gaps with external things, but they never satisfied me for long. The emptiness I felt couldn't be filled with more doing, more having. It required a return inward—to my own gifts, my own values, my own essence.

As the Dalai Lama so wisely said, "Man sacrifices his health to make money. Then he sacrifices his money to treat the disease. He is so anxious about the future that he does not enjoy the present, with the result that he does not live either in the present or the future. He lives as if he is never going to die—and then dies having never really lived."

A meaningful life requires intentional focus. Things of greater value often require more investment. A diamond, after all, is not as easily acquired as a cubic zirconia. The same applies to purpose. If I want a life that feels valuable and rich in meaning, I must prioritise what truly matters. That might mean releasing other things. Sacrifice, when done consciously, becomes an act of love.

Knowing what I am giving my life to—what I'm investing in—helps me live with appreciation and clarity. Without purpose, life can feel empty. But when I give my energy to the right things, life feels rich with meaning.

Carl Jung once said that purpose is found not through the pursuit of external desire, but through voluntary self-sacrifice. And I see that every day—in parents, caregivers, volunteers, and quiet acts of kindness. To love is to give. To serve is to live with purpose.

My truest nature is to love and be of service. And to live that way, I must keep returning to presence. Not the busy kind of doing—but the still, strong centre of being. The part of me that is whole, and already enough.

THE POWER OF PRESENCE

When I am deeply connected to the present moment, I find it easier to focus on what truly matters. This clarity of mind helps me identify my values, passions, and goals. By aligning my actions with these inner truths, I can make intentional choices that feel authentic and meaningful. For example, when I'm coaching others during health sessions, I sense that I'm contributing positively to their lives while also strengthening my own commitment to education, health, and connection. This brings a deep sense of fulfillment and satisfaction.

When I am mindful of each moment, the pace of life seems to slow. I notice more of what's happening around me and can make conscious decisions that influence outcomes in a positive way.

I remember a time when I was presenting to a large audience. I became aware of many pairs of eyes watching me. As my heart rate increased and anxiety began to build, I gently reminded myself to return to the present—feeling my feet firmly on the floor, slowing my speech, and speaking from my heart.

This shift helped me connect with the audience and the message I wanted to share. I wanted to express my passion, my values, and my truth. Being grounded in the moment gave me the clarity and calm to speak with intention and sincerity.

Presence also fosters authenticity and integrity. It encourages me to act in ways that reflect my true self. Living authentically allows me to pursue my purpose openly and make meaningful contributions to the world around me, in ways that feel aligned with who I am.

One of the most powerful examples of this was during a recent workshop I ran for women navigating midlife changes. I had notes prepared, but I felt called to speak from the heart instead. I let go of the script and trusted the connection in the room. What followed was one of the most moving sessions I've ever experienced. Women opened up, shared their truths, and leaned into the space we'd created together. It reminded me that when I show up fully, others feel safe to do the same.

Engaging in life with passion fuels my dedication and resilience, helping me overcome obstacles with grace and adaptability. Staying attuned to myself also deepens my sense of gratitude—for the people, experiences, and connections in my life. That gratitude nurtures a feeling of belonging and reminds me that our life journeys are connected.

Developing presence means moving from a state of thinking into a state of feeling. I ground myself in my physical body by becoming aware of the sensation of being "in my skin"—from the top of my head to the soles of my feet. From this physical awareness, I then visualise energy flowing from the crown of my head, through my body, and down into the earth.

When I notice areas that feel depleted or tense, I draw energy from the space around me—above, beside, or below—to fill those areas until they overflow. I then imagine sending any excess energy gently back to its source.

Presence is more than just physical awareness. It is an energetic state, powerful in both giving and receiving—much like my breath.

It's comforting to know this energy is universal and accessible to all of us. We each have the power to tap into it, and to use it for healing, growth, and connection.

THE ALCHEMY OF DESIRE

I'm not talking about the desire for materialistic things, like a new car, a holiday, or a new home. Desire, in its purest form, isn't driven by ego. It doesn't shout. It doesn't demand. It stirs quietly beneath the surface, whispering reminders of what could be possible if we only trusted ourselves enough to follow. These longings often arise not from emptiness, but from fullness—an overflow of love, of creativity, of life wanting to move through us in some new way.

I now see desire as a form of spiritual intelligence. A frequency that pulses beneath logic and reason, often defying timelines and expectations. Could it be the soul's way of saying, *"This matters. This is part of why you're here"*?

But desire is rarely neat. It brings with it vulnerability. It disrupts comfort. It asks us to risk being seen—not just by others, but by ourselves. It dares us to let go of who we think we "should" be so we can move toward who we truly are. And that is where the alchemy begins.

There was a moment in my own journey when I felt a quiet but persistent longing to step away from familiar security and explore a more creative, heart-led path. I had no plan, just a sense that there was more of me waiting to be expressed. At first, I ignored it, telling myself I should be grateful for what I had. But desire doesn't disappear when dismissed—it deepens. It started speaking through restlessness and quiet dissatisfaction. When I finally listened, it marked the beginning of a shift—from surviving to expressing, from structure to fluidity.

To transmute desire into something life-giving, we must meet it with honesty. Not all desire points to alignment—some arises from what we don't want: fear, rejection, pain. But the desire that lingers, that softens us when we lean into it, that stirs the heart more than the mind—that kind of desire is worth listening to.

When we follow that thread, something transforms. Our longings become less about acquiring and more about expressing. Less about chasing and more about allowing. We stop reaching for things outside of us and start awakening what's already within.

This is the alchemy: when we stop resisting our soul's true desires, they stop controlling us. They start shaping us. Guiding us. Softening us into deeper truth.

The more I've allowed desire to speak, the more I've realised it was never about getting more. It was about becoming more me.

LETTING LIFE MOVE THROUGH YOU

Desire may open the door, but surrender is what lets us walk through it.

There's a part of me that loves to plan, to predict, to make things happen. I've used discipline and drive to overcome countless challenges in life. But the further I walk this path, the more I realise that control, while comforting, often comes at the cost of peace. It narrows the channel through which life can flow.

Letting life move through you isn't about giving up. It's about softening the grip. About loosening the need to micromanage every outcome and instead opening to the idea that life is happening *with* you. That your body, your emotions, your intuition, your timing, your circumstance—they're all messengers, not obstacles.

We resist life most when it doesn't go to plan. When we get what we don't want, or don't get what we want. When the timing is off, when the outcome shifts, when we feel exposed or uncertain. But what if those moments aren't missteps? What if they are invitations—sacred pauses asking us to lean in, to let go, to trust?

This is not a passive surrender. It's an *active allowing*. A conscious decision to work with life's current rather than against it. It takes discernment. Courage. A willingness to listen deeply—even when what we hear isn't what we hoped for.

I've come to understand that alignment isn't created by effort alone. It emerges when we stop pushing against reality and start responding with presence. When we allow ourselves to be moved—not in a direction we control, but in one that reflects our truth.

Letting life move through you feels different. There's more breath. More space. More flow. You notice the synchronicities, the softness, the ease that comes when you're not gripping so tightly. And often, the very thing you were trying to force arrives once you've stopped chasing it.

There's a rhythm to this universe—a wisdom in its unfolding. When we honour that rhythm instead of overriding it, we begin to participate in life, not just manage it. We don't abandon action—but our actions arise from a deeper place. A place of clarity, not control. A place of trust.

This, too, is purpose: not just doing something meaningful, but *being someone surrendered*. Someone who allows life to move through them—freely, fully, and with grace.

DNA WITH A PURPOSE

Working out my purpose might feel like a big task—discovering the reason why I am here on earth. Yet, living a purposeful life might be simpler than I realise. For me, understanding what I'm here to do involves looking closely at why I was born into this body, with the genetics I inherited and the environment I grew up in.

I believe we are equipped with the tools and resources needed to fulfill our purpose. My unique biological make-up and the environment I was born into all provide what I need. It's a matter of learning to lean into our strengths and appreciate our vulnerabilities. These might be the clues to unlocking that purpose. By being authentic and mindful, breaking the habit of overthinking, coming from a heart-centred space, and deepening my understanding of who I am and why I do what I do—rooted in the quiet desires that rise from within rather than expectations placed upon me—I can awaken to what I am here to do—and how.

Living with intent means making conscious choices that reflect who I am and how I want to experience life. I want to feel empowered—not just by what I do, but by *why* I do it. Over time, I've noticed that the decisions I make are often influenced by how I feel in a given moment—those subtle emotional signals that rise up before thought. These emotions are shaped by everything from my biology to my environment, and they colour how I interpret what's happening around me. The same event can feel completely different depending on what state I'm in. That's why self-awareness matters so much. I might not be able to control every circumstance, but I've learned that I can shape how I respond—and that alone changes everything.

Another important area where my genetics and environment intersect is in relationships. The connections I have with myself and with others deeply shape my sense of purpose. Relationships with family, friends, mentors, and even strangers provide support, inspiration, and opportunities for growth. Love and kindness rank high on my values list. I feel that the interplay of hormones like adrenaline and oxytocin, combined with my Catholic upbringing, has drawn me toward situations and people that help me build caring connections. My actions affect others, and theirs affect me. Understanding how each contributes to our collective wellbeing is a powerful motivator in defining purpose. It reminds me that purpose is not something I must force—it is something I allow, through presence, openness, and trust.

Reflecting on pivotal and challenging moments also reveals their role in shaping my purpose. Sometimes, while in the midst of an experience, I don't see its significance. It's only in hindsight that I make the connection. As the eldest of four girls, I was placed in a role that required teaching, guiding, and nurturing. At times, the responsibility felt heavy, but I now see how this prepared me to be a responsible leader.

Reflecting on my interests and passions gives me insight into what makes me feel good and what brings meaning to my life. My career choices—neonatal nursing, personal training, health coaching—and my family's health challenges offered opportunities to explore nutrition, epigenetics, and functional medicine. These aren't just activities I enjoy; they're values I hold. Because I've spent time cultivating these passions, I've developed skills in these areas. These strengths have allowed me to impact both my own life and the lives of others. I have enough evidence to believe part of my purpose is to teach what I've learned about health and wellbeing—and I feel well placed to continue living this out.

Perhaps you have noticed similar turning points in your life that have guided your journey and sense of purpose?

The path to discovering and living my purpose isn't always straightforward. Following my passions and strengths brings joy, but growth often comes through challenges. Learning from failures gives me chances to try again. Resilience in adversity strengthens my commitment to becoming my best self. Living authentically and aligning my actions with my values can be difficult—especially when interacting with people who hold different beliefs or expectations. The depth of my commitment reveals what truly matters to me. True purpose often emerges when I live in harmony with my deepest convictions, and those convictions are tested.

It's also important to recognise that purpose is not static. As I evolve, so do my intentions. At some point, leaving a legacy might become part of my mission. I hope I've taught my sons, my husband, and all those I've had the privilege to live or work with something about understanding themselves. My wish is that they discover self-compassion and the ability to surrender to the higher power that unites us all. Leaving a legacy, to me, isn't about something obvious or tangible a thousand years from now. It's about impacting those around me now, so they, in turn, can inspire others—a continually evolving relationship with each other and the world.

I encourage you to explore, reflect, and grow as you deepen your own sense of purpose. Be open to different perspectives. Draw from your own experiences as a source of wisdom. And most importantly, cherish each moment with the intention of sharing your best self—helping to bring out the best in others. Together, we can shape a more beautiful world—one lived in harmony with who we are and how life flows through us.

Finding a bigger purpose isn't about uncovering a single, grand answer. It's more like unfolding a gentle journey—one that invites us to slow down, to listen deeply, and to be present with who we truly are in this moment. It's about embracing both our strengths and our vulnerabilities with kindness and allowing our desires—not just our skills—to guide us toward what matters most.

We may not always know where the path leads. But when we soften our resistance, when we stop trying to force outcomes and instead let life move through us, we begin to experience a quieter kind of knowing. A purpose that isn't defined by doing, but by being. That isn't static, but responsive and alive.

As I continue to evolve, so too does my purpose. Each chapter I live offers another opportunity to realign with what feels authentic. And in that realignment, I discover not just what I'm here to do—but how I'm here to love, serve, and grow.

Purpose is not a single path or final destination, but a conversation—a dialogue between our biology, our values, and a living, breathing expression of who we are becoming. We've examined how desire acts as a spiritual compass, how resistance points us toward inner work, and how surrender helps life move through us with greater ease. Purpose, then, is not just about what we do; it's about how we feel, how we connect, and how we respond.

You don't need to wait for a grand revelation. Every time you follow a quiet nudge, make a choice that reflects your values, or soften into the moment rather than control it, you are already living your purpose.

And now, with this deeper awareness, we begin to move from insight into creation. In the next chapter, we step into conscious design—how to take this inner knowing and begin shaping a life that reflects the truth of who you are.

Chapter Highlights

Life is the Present:
Busy-ness often masks our awareness of life as a precious gift.

The Power of Presence:
Moving from a thinking to a feeling state helps cultivate true presence. Presence is more than mindfulness; it's an embodied, heart-centred connection.

The Alchemy of Desire:
Authentic longing often points us toward soul-aligned purpose.

Letting Life Move Through You:
Living in flow doesn't mean life is easy; it means you're not constantly fighting it.

DNA with a Purpose:
Understanding one's genetics and environment reveals innate strengths which equip us with the resources we need to fulfill our unique purpose.

REFLECTIVE QUESTIONS

1. In what ways do you use breath or mindfulness to anchor yourself in the present?
   _____
   _____

2. What helps you move from simply thinking about your experiences to truly feeling them?
   _____
   _____

3. Can you distinguish between a desire driven by ego and one that comes from a deeper, more soulful place?
   _____
   _____

4. If you allowed your deepest desire to guide you for one day, what might you do differently?
   _____
   _____

5. Where in your life are you currently feeling resistance? What might that resistance be protecting?
   _____
   _____

6. How has your sense of purpose evolved over time, and what might it look like going forward?
   _____
   _____

7. What strengths and vulnerabilities have you noticed in yourself that might point toward your purpose?
   _____
   _____

THE BELIEF SHIFT

Chapter 9

CREATING WHAT'S NEXT

"And suddenly you know: it's time to start something new and trust the magic of beginnings."

MEISTER ECKHART

CREATING WHAT'S NEXT

There comes a moment—often quietly—when we begin to sense we're ready for something new. Not because we're incomplete, but because something within us has grown too big to stay where we are. It's not always a dramatic shift. Sometimes, it's as subtle as a gentle nudge inviting us to step more fully into life and co-create the next stage that is calling us.

As I reflect on the journey that brought me here—through awakening, alignment, and uncovering a bigger purpose—I feel something stirring. Not a restless need to chase or prove, but a grounded desire to shape what comes next with intention and heart.

This season of life feels different. There's less striving and more sensing. Less forcing and more flowing. I no longer crave a rigid five-year plan or a list of grand achievements. Instead, I want to co-create from a place of alignment. I want to listen more closely to what life is asking of me and offer my gifts with both courage and care.

Creating what's next isn't about fixing what's broken or reinventing who we are. It's about expanding into who we're becoming. It's about honouring our growth, values, and desires—and allowing that deeper knowing to shape how we move forward.

Of course, stepping into something new often comes with uncertainty. We may question if we're ready. We may worry about getting it wrong. Doubts we thought we'd outgrown can creep back in. But these doubts don't mean we're unprepared. They simply remind us that we're about to do something meaningful.

If you're standing at the edge of a new beginning—whether it's a career change, a creative dream, a healing path, or simply a different way of being—I hope this chapter reconnects you with what matters most. What are you ready to feel more of? What are you ready to release? What truth is asking to be lived more fully through you?

Life is a series of choices. I am where I am now because of the choices I've made, the beliefs I've held, and the actions I've taken. But now, as an empowered and aware adult, I can choose again. I can let go of what no longer fits and step forward with clarity and care.

That doesn't mean it's always easy. Old thought loops—those familiar, unconscious patterns—can hold us back. Some mornings,

I catch myself going through the motions: making breakfast without tasting it, rushing through the day without noticing the sky, waiting for it all to be over. That's not creation. That's survival.

To consciously create my life, I have to interrupt autopilot. I have to notice the mental playlist that's playing beneath the surface. I don't need to silence my thoughts, but I do need to discern which ones I give power to.

Creation is energetic. What I build will always carry the frequency I bring to it. When I create from love, trust, and joy, the results reflect that. And sometimes, creation isn't about adding something new—it's about subtracting what no longer fits. Letting go. Clearing space. Chiselling truth from the excess.

My future can be a blank canvas—or a sculpture waiting to be revealed. Perhaps it will be both.

This chapter is your invitation to create what's next—not from pressure but from the quiet wisdom of your heart. When you unplug from the noisy mind and return to the source of your most loving self, you reconnect with your power. You choose how you want to feel. What you want to experience. What you want to offer. Who you want to become.

DISRUPTING THE DEFAULT

Writing this subheading reminded me of *The Matrix* movie series. For those unfamiliar, the story explores a battle between humans and artificial intelligence. The AI feeds a virtual reality into the minds of humans, convincing them that what they see is real. But a few people awaken to the truth and disrupt the illusion of the default reality. Their world is completely different.

In many ways, I've lived a similar metaphor. The information I take in shapes my beliefs, which then shape my perception of reality. Most of the time, I react without questioning where that information is coming from. But I've learned that I can choose to wake up. I can begin to ask: *"Where is this coming from? Is this true for me? Is this fear or love?"*

Like in the movie, some people don't know another reality is possible. They're so entwined in the story of their lives that they can't imagine it being different. I've been there too. It's not until we question the source and "unplug" that we realise a more aligned and fulfilling life is within reach.

As someone who lives a lot in her head, disconnecting from programmed mental chatter hasn't been easy. I still catch myself running loops of overthinking, self-doubt, or perfectionism. But now, I pause and ask: *"What is powering this thought? Is this helpful? Is this coming from a place of truth and love, or fear and habit?"* Bit by bit, with practice, I've trained myself to be more present, more conscious, and more self-compassionate.

This doesn't mean I've silenced all thoughts. But I've stopped trying to fight or suppress them. I let them rise and fall like waves. I watch them play out without being swept away. I see them like little children—loud, persistent, and attention-seeking—but ultimately, they settle when given space.

Being physically active helps me shift attention from my mind to my body. When I'm moving, I feel more present, more alive. My energy lifts, my spirit opens. I've noticed that when I'm in a high-energy, loving state, I feel expressive and connected. When I'm in a low-energy, fearful state, I feel withdrawn and small. So instead of trying to think my way out of it, I move.

Sometimes it's not about dissecting every emotion or unearthing every belief. Sometimes it's as simple as recognising the results I'm getting in life and tracing them back to how I'm feeling and behaving. If I'm flat and unmotivated, I move. If I'm distracted, I ask myself what I'm avoiding. If I'm feeling good, I celebrate it—and use that energy to create something beautiful.

This is how I unplug. Gently. Lovingly. Repeatedly. And each time I do, I reconnect to something real. Something true. Something that brings me back to life.

LIVING BY DESIGN

I know now that my current reality has been shaped by the beliefs I've held in the past. As Henry Ford said, "Whether you think you can, or you think you can't—you're right." My life today reflects what I once believed was possible. But that doesn't mean I'm stuck. Each present moment holds the power to shift course. I can begin again—gently, intentionally.

While I can't change what's happened, I can choose the meaning I assign to it. And that shift in meaning can transform my story. When I interpret old experiences through a more compassionate and empowered lens, I loosen the grip of limiting beliefs and begin to build new, supportive ones. For instance, where I once believed that perfection was necessary, I now believe that being real is far more powerful—and far more liberating.

Negative emotions, misaligned outcomes, or critical inner chatter aren't signs that I've failed—they're invitations. They show me I've slipped into an old pattern that no longer fits. They prompt me to ask better questions, like: *"What would I need to believe to feel better right now?"* From that space of inquiry, I can create a new response, one rooted in awareness and choice.

This is the power of presence. When I'm fully engaged in the now—not replaying the past or worrying about the future—I have access to my deepest wisdom. I can choose thoughts, beliefs, and behaviours that reflect the life I want to create. And I can do it from a place of calm, clarity, and courage.

Letting go of the need for things to be perfect has been a turning point. For years, I believed I had to work harder, be better, achieve more. But perfection is an illusion. It kept me focused on lack, not possibility. These days, I value progress over perfection. I aim to do my best—but with grace, not pressure.

Creating a life I love means getting radically honest about what nourishes me—and what depletes me. It means listening to the whisper beneath the noise, breathing before I say yes, and asking, *"Is this true for me?"* Sometimes, it means removing instead of adding. Saying no. Creating boundaries.

This is the work of living by design: making conscious choices that align with my values, desires, and truth. Not once, but over and over again. Staying true to myself is a daily practice—a sacred, tender rebellion in a world that profits from our disconnection.

But when I do, something beautiful happens. Life becomes less about performing and more about participating. I stop existing by default and start creating by intention. I align from the inside out. I soften instead of striving. I root myself in what's real. And from that place, I begin to design what's next—not just with my mind, but with my heart.

TRUSTING THE SLOW MAGIC OF BECOMING

After designing a life rooted in truth and intention, the next step is learning to live it—moment by moment—with patience and presence. Bringing a vision into reality isn't about overnight transformation. It's about honouring the slow magic of becoming. That kind of growth doesn't always look spectacular on the surface. Often, it's quiet. Subtle. Unfolding in the background, reshaping us from within.

Throughout this book, I've shared how I've come to better understand who I am and why. Yes, I am the result of my upbringing, biology, and the meaning I've made of my experiences—but I'm not defined by those alone. I am more than my past. And so are you.

To create a life that feels aligned and deeply fulfilling, we must become clear on what we truly desire. That clarity becomes our compass. But desire alone isn't enough. Along the way, we'll meet resistance in the form of old habits, unconscious fears, outdated beliefs, and external distractions. Living with intention means learning to meet those edges with compassion rather than judgment.

Like any meaningful creation, a life we love takes time. We need space to gather, mix, rest, and refine. Just as a seed becomes a tree through seasons of unseen growth, our transformation often happens below the surface. Even when progress feels slow or invisible, trust is key. We keep tending to the vision. We keep showing up.

I often check in with myself, not out of pressure, but as a way of staying attuned: *"How am I feeling? What am I believing? What are my actions revealing about the life I'm creating?"* These questions bring me back to presence. They help me course-correct with gentleness, not criticism.

I've come to trust that timing has its own wisdom. Just like pregnancy can't be rushed, or a flower won't bloom before it's ready, our lives unfold in a rhythm that doesn't always match our expectations—but often exceeds them in richness and meaning when we allow the process to unfold.

The key is to create from love, not fear. To make choices not because we should, but because they feel aligned. To let gratitude soften the start of each day and presence guide what follows. When I pause to appreciate my body, my family, my breath—I signal to life: *I'm ready. Let's co-create.*

Of course, the path isn't always smooth. There are detours, delays, and days of doubt. But when my vision is rooted in love—when it's truly mine, not borrowed or inherited—I find the strength to keep going. Even when things don't go to plan, I can meet them with an open heart and trust that something meaningful is still unfolding.

To live through love is to lead from the heart. It's not about perfection—it's about presence. It's about showing up as we are, embracing both the uncertainty and the sacredness of becoming. With practice, with trust, with heart-led presence, something new takes root. A deeper knowing. A quiet courage. A readiness to walk forward—not on a path prescribed by others, but one we are co-creating with each mindful step.

A NEW PATH EMERGING

Ahead of me lies the surprise of yet-undiscovered experiences—of unknown time, shape, and rhythm. Endless possibilities are waiting to unfold. The path is made up of unfamiliar turns, unpredictable moments, and evolving chapters—for the journey itself, and for the one walking it.

Activating my capacity for growth and authentic alignment on these new or dissolving paths is an invitation. A chance to explore and redefine who I am—moment by moment. I am not defined by my past, nor confined by the labels I've carried. I am a masterpiece in progress, with the power to uncover and embody the truth of who I really am.

Becoming who I am today has been—and continues to be—a process. It takes conscious choice, compassionate curiosity, and the willingness to examine what thoughts, feelings, and behaviours are ready to shift. As I move forward, I carry the light of awareness with me, gently illuminating the hidden habits that no longer serve. It can be messy, and that's okay. I no longer need to "fit in." Life doesn't need to be neat or polished to be meaningful.

There's no rulebook. No linear route. The journey is spiral, seasonal, and deeply personal. While I believe there is a destination—rooted in love, truth, and purpose—there's no fixed timeline or predetermined path to reach it. I am exactly where I need to be. And so are you.

That doesn't mean everything feels clear or easy. It means this moment—however messy, uncertain, or in-between—is part of the path. It's not a detour. It's a doorway. Even when we feel lost or stuck, we are being invited to pause, listen, and learn something essential.

Being exactly where we need to be is not about comfort or certainty—it's about presence. It's trusting that what's unfolding has meaning, even if we can't yet see the whole picture. It reminds us that growth isn't always visible, and healing rarely happens on a deadline.

So if you're questioning, doubting, or still figuring things out—you're not behind. You're in process. And that's a sacred place to be.

For much of my life, my decisions were guided by logic, analysis, and a mind constantly in motion. It led to a lot of busy doing. But with time, I've come to trust a deeper kind of wisdom—one that doesn't shout or strategise but quietly leads from the heart. When I let my heart become the conductor of the orchestra, everything starts to fall into harmony.

I now ask myself questions like: *"What would love do here?"* or *"What might be possible if I gave myself full permission to believe that the best is on its way?"* These questions unlock something beyond intellect—they tap into the intelligence of the spirit, the body, and the soul. The answers that arise are wiser than anything I could reason into existence. There's a powerful energy that speaks more clearly than the voice of doubt. And I've learned to listen.

One of the greatest tools for quieting the noise and tuning into this guidance has been daily meditation. Just a few intentional minutes of stillness each day can recalibrate my entire internal state. In the stillness, I can hear where the music is off-key. I can sense what needs refining—whether it's the rhythm, the tone, the melody, or the pitch. Like composing a new song, each note matters.

Sometimes the old music still plays: the familiar tune of not good enough, not ready yet, or what if it goes wrong? But now, I can hear a new melody rising beneath it—one that says, you are more than enough, you are ready, and good things are coming.

Becoming aware of the background music we've unknowingly played for years is what allows us to rewrite it. And when we do, we open the door to a new dance—one that feels true, liberating, and beautifully our own.

As this chapter draws to a close, I'm reminded that every ending is also a beginning. Creating what's next isn't about having everything perfectly mapped out. It's about tuning into what feels real, what makes us come alive, and what allows us to move through the world with greater awareness, intention, and love.

The practices I've shared—disrupting unconscious patterns, choosing aligned beliefs, trusting life's timing, and following the heart—are not a one-time fix, but a lifelong rhythm. One step at a time, one breath at a time, we continue returning to what matters most. We learn to embrace both the certainty of our inner truth and the uncertainty of what lies ahead.

There is power in letting go. Power in starting again. Power in choosing to live a life that feels like your own. Whatever your path may look like, may it be one of your choosing—lit by self-compassion and guided by the quiet wisdom within.

You don't need to have everything figured out to begin again.

Creating what's next is not about chasing an ideal version of yourself—it's about honouring who you are now and allowing that truth to shape what unfolds. The life you're longing to live may not require a radical reinvention, but a gentle re-alignment—an invitation to walk forward with more intention, trust, and love.

There will always be uncertainty. The mind may hesitate. The path may curve. But when you learn to listen to your inner wisdom, let go of outdated beliefs, and follow the quiet pull of your heart, the next chapter begins to write itself.

Each moment offers a choice: to repeat the familiar, or to create something new.

You are the author of what comes next. You get to choose what to carry forward, what to release, and how to show up. You get to design a life that reflects your values, your growth, your vision, and your essence.

There's no need to rush. Life will meet you exactly where you are.

Trust the slow magic of becoming. Trust the quiet unfolding of your path. And most of all, trust yourself.

Chapter Highlights

Disrupting the Default:
The stories we unconsciously live by are often inherited or fear-based—until we wake up and question them.

Living By Design:
Our present is shaped by past beliefs, but we are free to choose differently now. A life we love is built from self-acceptance, alignment, and daily conscious choices.

Trusting the Slow Magic of Becoming:
Creating a fulfilling life takes vision, patience, and a willingness to evolve. Life's timing is often wiser than our planning—trust the rhythm, not just the results.

A New Path Emerging:
Your path is unique, evolving, and co-created with each moment of awareness.

REFLECTIVE QUESTIONS

1. What beliefs or stories have you been living by on autopilot—and are they still serving you?

2. How do you typically respond when you feel caught in overthinking or fear? What helps you shift?

3. What past patterns are you ready to interrupt so you can create new results?

4. What's one belief you could release today that would create more spaciousness and freedom in your life?

5. Where in your life are you being asked to trust the slow unfolding of something meaningful?

6. How do you reconnect with your body or inner wisdom when you're feeling stuck or unclear?

7. What does it look like to walk your own path with love, courage, and truth?

THE BELIEF SHIFT

Chapter 10

INTEGRATION – A LIFE REWRITTEN

"Believe in yourself and all that you are. Know that there is something inside you that is greater than any obstacle."

CHRISTIAN D. LARSON

Well done for arriving here. You are so close to the end of this book, and perhaps the beginning of a new chapter within yourself. Whether you've read every word or skimmed a few pages, the fact that you're still here speaks volumes. It means you've been willing to look within. To reflect. To grow. And that alone is something to celebrate.

But let's be clear—this is not the end. Not for you. You are still becoming. As long as life moves through you, there will be new moments to meet, new challenges to navigate, and new truths to uncover. You are always evolving.

The journey of rewriting your inner story is not a straight line. It's layered and alive, shaped by awareness, reflection, disruption, and healing. Even after deep transformation, there will still be days that stretch you. Let them. Let every challenge be a reminder of your resilience, not a reason to retreat.

You've walked through stories shaped by your past. You've questioned beliefs that once defined you. You've explored identity, purpose, desire, and truth. And now, you stand here—not at the finish line, but at a powerful threshold: the doorway to integration.

This chapter is about bringing it all together. About moving from *knowing* to *being*. About living each day not just as someone who has read about transformation—but as someone who embodies it. Integration means your beliefs, thoughts, feelings, and actions increasingly reflect the truth of who you are.

It's not about becoming someone else. It's about becoming more fully yourself—anchored, aware, and alive. You don't need to chase a shinier version of you. You're not here to strive endlessly for improvement. You're here to remember your wholeness. As the Hindu sage Ramana Maharshi wrote, "You are already that which you seek." Let that be both comfort and compass.

So as we move into this chapter, I invite you to pause—not to evaluate how far you've come, but to feel where you are right now. Grounded in this moment. Open to what's next. And ready to live from the inside out.

Because the real shift—the belief shift—is not just about believing differently. It's about living differently. And that begins with a powerful decision.

YOUR MISSION, IF YOU CHOOSE TO ACCEPT IT

Wherever you are right now is perfectly okay. You don't need to fix or change anything unless you choose to. You are not broken. You are not behind. You are not incomplete. You are already whole, already enough.

And yet—within you is an abundant source of energy waiting to be remembered, reclaimed, and shared. It's not something you need to create. It's something you uncover. A quiet light that's been there all along. Over time, you may even come to realise that you *are* that light. And the more you live from it, the more others around you benefit too.

To shift from identifying with your thoughts and emotions to simply being aware of them requires a deep and intentional pause. We are not our thoughts. Not our feelings. Not even our behaviours. We are the ones who *see* these things. We are the awareness beneath them all—the consciousness behind the experience.

As I've shared earlier, I still catch myself at times defining who I am by what I do. It's familiar and easy for the mind to cling to identities—roles, titles, expectations. They give us a structure for belonging. But they are not the full story. You are so much more than any label you've worn.

You are not your job. Not your body. Not your mind. These are things you *have*—not who you *are*. Beneath them is a quiet, steady presence that watches and witnesses without judgement. That essence is your true self. It remains stable, even when life feels messy.

I often think of it like the ocean. On the surface, the waves may crash with noise and urgency. But deep below, the water is still. Calm. Unmoved. That same stillness exists within you. It's not the fleeting peace that depends on things going your way, but a deep peace that simply *is*—independent of circumstance. That is the peace we all long for. And it's already yours.

When we shift our attention from the choppy surface to the calm beneath, life feels different. We stop clinging. We start flowing. Control loosens its grip. The burden lifts. And slowly, we remember: our natural state is lightness, not struggle. Freedom, not fear.

Yes, there will still be stormy days. Life will never be without challenge. But you can learn to ride the waves. To release the urge to fight the current and move with life instead of against it. And with time, even the rough waters become teachers. They shape you. Strengthen you. And when the sun returns, you receive it with new appreciation—because you've earned the stillness through the storm.

When life doesn't unfold the way I hoped, I remind myself: *"It happened the only way it could have"*. If something else were meant to happen, it would have. This doesn't mean we stop caring. It means we stop resisting. We soften into what is. Every experience becomes an invitation to witness, to reflect, to grow.

At the start of this book, I was searching. For answers. For understanding. For reasons. I asked: *"Why am I like this? Why did this happen? Why do I feel this way?"* But sometimes *why* is the wrong question. Perhaps it's not about a question at all.

What if life isn't meant to be figured out, but felt? What if the invitation is not to live in our heads—but to live from the heart? What if we stopped chasing meaning and started trusting. What if it was about being rather than doing? An experience rather than a mystery to solve?

Yes, our past matters. Our biology, upbringing, and environment have shaped us. But they don't define us. The moment we become aware of the story, we gain the power to change it. We don't need to solve everything. We can meet the moment—not as a problem to solve, but as a gift to experience.

And that, perhaps, is your mission.

To live awake.
To bring your presence to the moment.
To respond with compassion.
To lead with love.

To be a conscious, grounded, healing force in a world that needs exactly what you offer.

Not because you have to.

But because you can.

When we soften into what is, we make room for what's possible. We allow the next stage of our transformation to unfold—not through control, but through trust.

And when we begin to live this way—not perfectly, but consciously—we can't help but change. It happens quietly at first. But over time, the shift becomes undeniable.

YOU ARE FOREVER CHANGED

Experiences shape the very function of our cells. Even from the start of this book to now, something in you has shifted. Your thoughts, your feelings—your perspective—are no longer the same. Life may now be seen through a more expansive lens, one that filters out the noise and drama and offers space to respond instead of reacting. You're no longer swept away so easily. A new awareness has emerged—one that invites alignment with the wiser, more loving version of who you truly are.

I hope you've begun to recognise the creative power within you, and with it, a deeper sense of agency. This isn't about controlling life but about cultivating an inner and outer environment for growth. It's about releasing resistance—the static that disrupts the natural flow of your energy—and instead tuning into the calm vibrancy that's always been yours.

Perhaps you've discovered a new anchor point: a place within yourself that feels peaceful, steady, and real. Even when the mind spins or the body feels unsettled, there is stillness beneath it all. A knowing presence that whispers, *you are okay*. You've come to understand that doing more isn't always the answer. Sometimes, the solution is found in the quiet art of simply being.

It is in this presence—in this stillness—that I've become open to the transformative truths of love, healing, and personal evolution. I've come to see that the waters of life run deep. On the surface, things can feel turbulent and chaotic. Shallow waters are easily disrupted by rocks, debris, and noise. But the deeper the current, the less it is disturbed. Superficial living—focused on appearances, perfection, or performance—tends to agitate the soul. But living through love returns me to my depth. It allows me to create from truth, not fear.

The challenge now is to build sustainable, aligned habits that support the vision of the life you desire. That vision isn't a fantasy—it's a reality waiting to unfold through consistent intention. For many years, I looked for peace and fulfillment in all the wrong places, thinking I just needed to figure it out. But no matter how hard you search in the wrong place, you won't find what you're looking for. Like searching for keys outside when you lost them in the house or combing through your home for your child's jumper when it's still at school—sometimes we just need to look in the right direction.

For a long time, I tried to think my way into peace. I worked hard to replace negative thoughts with positive ones, to outsmart my inner critic. And while this helped at times, it was never consistent. The mind, after all, is restless. Buddhists call it the "monkey mind"—always jumping, always clinging, never fully still. Trying to quiet it by force is like trying to stop a river from flowing.

Sustainable change, I've learned, comes from something deeper than thought. It's rooted in awareness. There will be seasons when peace feels like a gentle breeze and others when it's harder to access—but it's always there, beneath the surface. You don't need a peaceful mind to experience peace. You just need to remember that peace lives *within* you, not beyond you.

Often, it's in our most uncomfortable moments that meaningful change becomes possible. Discomfort brings motivation. Resistance sparks questions. And questions lead to creation. When something no longer feels right, we are gifted an opportunity to make it better—not by fighting the moment, but by listening to what it's asking of us. The next step reveals itself when we let go of our resistance to it.

The changes you've made—whether internal or external—won't always be visible or measurable. But they are real. You'll know them by the way you speak, the choices you make, the energy you carry. When you're committed to living from love, discipline becomes devotion. As Craig Groeschel writes, "Discipline is choosing what you want most over what you want now." It's a daily decision to align your time, energy, and attention with what truly matters.

You'll still need your courage, your resilience, and your grace. Challenges will come, but now you have a foundation—a stillness within you that won't collapse under pressure. When the noise of the world rises, you can choose to turn down the volume and listen inwardly instead. You can choose to attend not to the chaos, but to the quiet.

I call this practice *emotional surfing*. It's a daily invitation to ride the waves of experience without losing yourself to them. It's not about controlling the ocean but learning to move with it. Some days are easier than others. But over time, I've learned to return more quickly and easily to my calm centre. It's not perfect—but it's powerful.

Still, I am not immune to reactivity. None of us are. That's why awareness matters. When emotions rise, the temptation to avoid or attach is strong. But I've found that when I stay present, allow the moment to pass through me, and soften my grip, something beautiful happens: I emerge wiser, freer, and more open to what's next.

My mind will always have something to say. It loves to advise, command, and critique. But I've learned not to listen to all of it. The heart, though—it speaks in energy, not in volume. It moves with grace, not resistance. The heart doesn't shout. It offers. It receives. It reminds me of who I really am.

Often, my mind and body will send mixed signals. That's okay. I can observe both with compassion and choose from a place of alignment. I don't need to fix everything. I can accept what is, and trust that every moment holds the potential for growth. Every moment is here because of all that came before it.

And now, you get to decide what comes next.

My ongoing mission is to notice when I'm seeking comfort as a shield from fear—and then, gently, to step into courage. To take the leap. To trust that life is always trying to express itself through me. The edge of change can feel vulnerable, uncertain, raw. But the growth is always worth it.

The lesson I continue to learn is this: resistance is often what holds us back—not the challenge itself. Resistance can look like avoidance, fear, control, or even force. We resist what we cannot control, and we cling to what we don't want to lose. But healing comes when we let go of the resistance to pain, the attachment to pleasure, and the illusion that life should be any other way than what we are experiencing.

It's okay to feel uncomfortable. It's okay to feel joy. It's okay to let things go.

Releasing resistance doesn't mean we won't feel fear, grief, or uncertainty. It means we no longer allow those emotions to stop us from moving forward. When we soften into what *is*, we make room for what's possible. We allow the next stage of our transformation to gently unfold.

Trust in the process extends not only to life itself, but also to the emotions that move through us. Emotions, after all, are part of that unfolding—if we let them flow.

EMOTION AS ENERGY IN MOTION

Feelings are meant to be transient. *E-motion* is, quite literally, energy in motion. As a form of energy, emotions are designed to move through us—not to be held onto or locked away.

Naturally, I want to hold onto feelings that are pleasurable. I might try to recreate a joyful experience to relive its warmth. On the other hand, I don't consciously want to keep negative emotions around. But if I haven't processed them properly, they can get stuck in my body. I might "lock" them away to avoid discomfort. The trouble is, they never really disappear. They eventually resurface—perhaps as pain, frustration, fatigue, or a quiet irritation that grows louder over time until I'm forced to pay attention. One way or another, the energy needs to move. It needs to be acknowledged, expressed, and released—*if* I want to live freely and vibrantly.

Becoming curious about what I'm feeling—and asking better questions—helps me name what's going on beneath the surface. When I do this, my mind will instinctively try to find a logical explanation or quick solution. Sometimes I'll be lucky enough to realise that the real problem isn't the emotion itself, but the *meaning* I've given to the experience.

Take loneliness, for example. Feeling alone doesn't automatically create pain. It's the *story* I attach to that feeling that can hurt— *"I'm not safe"*, *"I'm not loveable"*, *"No one wants to be with me"*, *"I must not be good enough"*. To escape that pain, I might turn to coping strategies: drinking, overeating, scrolling, overworking, isolating, numbing. But these strategies don't solve the root cause. They simply help me avoid the discomfort—temporarily.

We tend to reject lower-frequency emotions because they feel heavy, raw, or uncomfortable. But all emotions—whether pleasant or painful—are asking for one thing: our presence. They don't need to be fixed. They need to be felt.

Emotion is energy, and energy wants to move. Some emotions will repel, some will attract, and others will neutralise—but all of them want to flow. To support that, we don't need to over-analyse. We simply need to allow. We need to be present with the feeling and listen to what it's asking for. Sometimes, loneliness is just asking for companionship. Fear may be asking for safety. Sadness might be asking to be held—not pushed away.

Instead of resisting or numbing, we can meet our emotions with kindness. Rather than strategising how to escape a feeling, we can practice sitting with it. Let it be. Hold space for it. Let it pass through, wrapped in our own love, presence, and compassion.

Think of a time when someone close to you was grieving. They didn't want you to fix anything. They just wanted you there—to sit beside them, quietly and fully present. They wanted to feel held, not hurried. Our emotions want the same thing. They want us to notice, acknowledge, and accept them without trying to change them. When we allow our feelings to be seen and heard, they soften. They settle. They pass.

Emotions are meant to be temporary—unless we resist them. When we push them down or suppress them, they become stuck. But when we allow them, they move. This is how we create space. This is how we become more responsive and less reactive. And it begins with self-awareness—by taking an honest internal inventory and meeting ourselves with grace.

In today's world, the lines between our inner and outer realities have become so blurred that many of us have lost touch with authentic connection—not only with the world, but with ourselves. Yet it's possible to return. To remember. To reconnect.

We can peel back the layers and rediscover who we truly are—biologically, emotionally, mentally, psychologically, socially, and spiritually. We can reawaken our *felt* inner knowing and free ourselves from the endless loops of overthinking. We can surrender the need to solve and, instead, listen from the heart.

This is where the truth of who we are lives—not in the mind's chatter, but in the still space of trust. A trust in ourselves, in life, and in the invisible threads that weave it all together. When we align with this deeper truth, a new path begins to reveal itself. A path that is already within us—waiting patiently to be walked. Waiting to be expressed. Waiting to be lived.

To walk that path, we must also learn to step back—to observe the flow without being swept away. This is where real freedom lives: in the space between stimulus and response.

BECOMING THE OBSERVER OF YOUR LIFE

Have you ever noticed the distance that forms between you and what's happening when you simply sit back and watch something unfold—like observing a sports match rather than playing in it? You might care about the outcome, but you also know you can't change it. You're removed from the action. A similar dynamic occurs when you step back and become the observer of your own life. Instead of being swept up in drama or letting circumstances define you, you begin to shift the energy around what you're feeling—just by witnessing it.

This witnessing creates space. It allows you to hold difficult emotions without being consumed by them. You no longer have to resist or suppress them. Instead, you can allow them to rise, move, and eventually pass. It's only when we resist it that it becomes stuck or amplified.

One of the most powerful tools we have is the ability to shift our focus from the head to the heart. Rather than trying to think our way out of discomfort—grasping for solutions, rationalisations, or distractions—we can simply pause, breathe, and drop into the heart space. From this place, we're better able to feel, process, and release the energy moving through us.

As Michael A. Singer, author of *The Untethered Soul*, beautifully writes: "The mind is where the soul goes to hide from the heart." When we feel emotional discomfort, we often retreat into the mind. We distract ourselves with thoughts, analyse what's happening, or build stories around why we feel the way we do. But thinking rarely brings peace. It often delays healing. Until we've allowed ourselves to feel fully and completely, the energy remains—waiting for release.

Becoming the observer allows us to witness the energy of our experience without identifying with it. Instead of saying, *"I am angry"* or *"I am a bad person"*, we can say, *"I notice anger is present"*, or *"I'm having self-critical thoughts"*. This subtle shift helps loosen the grip of identity and allows space for self-compassion.

Because we're physical beings, we often assign form to our feelings. We might pin emotions on people, situations, the weather, or even our jobs. We cling to what feels good and resist what feels bad. But either way, we're still attaching. And attachment is what gives emotions their charge.

The gift of observation is that it softens attachment. It invites surrender—not in a passive way, but in a powerful, spacious way. We begin to notice the difference between what is happening (the situation) and how it feels (the experience). We understand that neither defines who we are. We are not our emotions or our thoughts. We are the awareness that sees them.

Returning to the heart space is a recurring invitation. It reminds us that we don't have to *do* anything about discomfort. We can simply *feel* it. When we allow energy to flow through us, it often dissolves on its own. The heart is incredibly intelligent. It senses, it expands, and it contracts. When we feel intense sadness or profound love, we instinctively hold our chest, not our head. We know, intuitively, that the heart is where our true emotional centre lives.

When the heart is closed, we feel it—a tightness, a heaviness. That's the sensation of blocked energy. But when the heart is open, energy flows. We feel lighter, freer, more expansive. This is our natural state, yet modern life often disrupts it. We move quickly. We overthink. We crowd our minds with noise and distraction. In doing so, we block the flow that would otherwise bring us back into balance.

These blocks come from within—our thoughts, our interpretations, our habits. The energy still tries to move, but our resistance holds it back. Thankfully, releasing that resistance doesn't require perfection. It simply requires presence. Allowing life to be as it is, without armouring ourselves against what we don't like, dissolves many of the internal walls we've built.

There is so much energy within us waiting to flow. And when we stop resisting, we begin to feel more peace—not because life has changed, but because *we have*. We've stepped into the role of observer. We've become the space in which all experience is allowed.

Integration isn't about getting it all right. It's about coming home to yourself—again and again. It's the practice of remembering what matters, even when the noise of the world pulls you in other directions. It's the return to presence when you've drifted into distraction, the softening of resistance when you'd rather run, and the quiet courage to live aligned with your truth, even when it feels vulnerable.

There's no finish line to this work. And that's not a failure—it's a gift. Because each new day is a chance to respond with love, to breathe into the unknown, to trust the unfolding. You'll still have doubts. You'll still forget. But you'll also remember more quickly. Realign more easily. And live more fully.

This is what it means to rewrite your life through awareness. Not by escaping discomfort, but by meeting it with presence. And not by becoming someone new, but by fully becoming who you already are.

You're not starting over. You're starting *from*. From wisdom. From wholeness. From love.

Keep walking. Keep trusting. Keep choosing.

Chapter Highlights

Your Mission, If You Choose to Accept It:
You are already whole, and nothing outside of you needs to be fixed for you to begin.

You Are Forever Changed:
Even subtle shifts in awareness change your biology, behaviour, and sense of agency.

Emotion as Energy in Motion:
Emotions are energy designed to move through you, not be suppressed or clung to.

Becoming the Observer of Your Life:
Observation creates space between stimulus and response, softening reactivity.

REFLECTIVE QUESTIONS

1. What part of you feels most aligned right now and how can you support that alignment in daily life?
   _____
   _____
   _____

2. Where are you still gripping, resisting, or trying to control and what might it feel like to soften instead?
   _____
   _____
   _____

3. What story are you ready to stop telling and what truth is rising in its place?
   _____
   _____
   _____

4. What would it look like for you to live awake not just in moments of insight, but in the rhythm of ordinary life?
   _____
   _____
   _____

5. What is your next small act of integration that honours who you've become?
   _____
   _____
   _____

Chapter 11

NOT THE FINAL CHAPTER, BUT A LIVING ENDING

"I am not what happened to me. I am what I choose to become."

CARL JUNG

NOT THE FINAL CHAPTER, BUT A LIVING ENDING

This chapter is here to remind you that the work isn't behind you. It's within you. This is not about closing the book. It's about living it forward.

You've gathered tools. You've softened into presence. You've shifted old beliefs and found new ways of seeing. But integration isn't a single act—it's a practice. It's how you show up when no one's watching. How you respond when fear tries to crawl back in. How you honour your truth when it would be easier to fall back into old patterns.

This chapter is not the end. It's an opening. A bridge between who you've been and who you're becoming. A moment to take stock, to trust what you now know, and to step with intention into your next chapter—whatever that may look like.

Let's begin by naming something that often gets overlooked on the path to personal growth: the real problem isn't what we think it is.

SEEING THE REAL PROBLEM

A big part of finding any real solution is being willing to look deeper—beyond the surface symptoms—to uncover the root cause of our unhappiness. It's easy to focus on what's obvious and call it "the problem". For example, someone might say they have a weight problem. But in many cases, weight isn't really the problem. There is something deeper.

The problem is the meaning we give to our experience, and more than that—what it says about us.

A "weight" problem is a problem because it triggers hidden subconscious beliefs such as: *"I am not lovable"*, *"I am not attractive"*, *"I am not worthy"* or *"I am not good enough"*. Unfortunately, the belief continues to amplify the symptom, and reactive behaviours contribute to the problem, making it a self-fulfilling prophecy.

What's really at the root is the narrative we build around the stories—the interpretations we create—that often lead to pain. Most of us haven't learned how to sit with difficult emotions in a healthy, regulated way. So instead, we avoid. We distract. We seek relief outside of ourselves. And in doing so, we suppress, or resist, the flow of emotion through us, as it's designed to do.

This creates a pattern: we move toward what feels good and away from what feels bad. On the surface, that might seem logical. But when our sense of peace depends on avoiding discomfort, we become increasingly dependent on external fixes—more food, more scrolling, more praise, more noise. And all the while, the original emotion—the fear, the grief, the anxiety, the unworthiness—remains unacknowledged.

What's really needed is a new kind of inquiry. Not, *"How can I make this feeling go away?"* but *"What is this experience asking of me?"*

Questions like:

- What meaning have I attached to this experience that might not be true?
- What am I really concerned about beneath the surface of this habit?
- What was I hoping to avoid or gain when I first started this behaviour?
- What is this discomfort pointing me towards?
- What belief is driving this action—and is it serving me?
- What do I truly need right now?

These are deep questions. And they require honesty, curiosity, and compassion.

Looking at my own life, I can now see how many of my habits were created to avoid discomfort and reach for something more pleasurable or affirming. For instance, it feels good to be skilled, respected, and needed in my work. That sense of usefulness once fed a strong identity—the belief that who I was could be measured by how well I performed or how much I contributed.

But over time, I've come to understand that what I *do* is not who I *am*. And while I still take pride in doing meaningful work, I now focus more on *how* I show up—bringing presence, heart, and authenticity to what I do, rather than letting the role itself define my worth.

Letting go of outdated identities, or even successful ones that no longer feel aligned, has been one of the most liberating and confronting aspects of growth. It has allowed space for something new to emerge—something more whole, more true.

Now, my ongoing mission is to recognise when I'm using comfort to hide from fear—and then gently choose courage instead. To take the leap. To trust that life is always seeking to express itself through me in new ways. And yes, that trust sometimes takes me to the edge of discomfort.

But I've come to see that discomfort isn't the enemy. Resistance is. The resistance to pain. The resistance to change. The resistance to what is.

When I release that resistance—even just a little—I return to the flow of life. I stop fighting. I stop trying to manipulate outcomes. And in that space, I feel free again. Not because everything is perfect, but because I'm no longer armoured against reality.

And that's how I've come to see the real problem—not as the external trigger or even the painful feeling, but the resistance to being with it. Once that softens, healing begins.

To release resistance, we must first understand what we're resisting—and more often than not, it's rooted in a belief we've never questioned. What if the real barrier isn't what's happening, but what we've come to believe about it?

BELIEVE IT. OR NOT

When I was a teenager, there was a television show called *Ripley's Believe It or Not?*—a documentary series that shared strange occurrences, unexplained mysteries, and unusual phenomena. Many of the stories seemed too far-fetched to be real, but apparently, they were true.

Our minds can be a bit like that show. They're constantly offering us stories and conclusions, wanting us to believe everything we "see" (believe, think, or feel) is absolute truth. Somewhere along the way—likely during our early years of conditioning—we absorbed meaning and formed beliefs that became the rules of our internal programming. The mind wants to be right. And it's clever, persuasive, and persistent. We follow its lead because it's familiar. Over time, these thoughts become automatic, rarely questioned, yet quietly running the show.

But what if we *did* question them?

What would you *rather* believe?

If we took a closer look, we'd likely find that many of our thoughts stem not from truth, but from assumptions, outdated conclusions, or imagined futures. Predictions that never came true. Stories based on fear. What if, instead of unconsciously accepting these mental narratives, we chose to believe something that served us?

We explored this in Chapter 3—how beliefs create thoughts and feelings that shape our behaviours. Understanding the origin of a belief can sometimes help, but it's not always necessary. What *is* essential is recognising whether we're still holding onto beliefs that limit us.

One way to do this is to observe the outcomes in our lives. Our results are often a mirror of our beliefs. Repeating patterns, poor outcomes, or feelings of being stuck are often symptoms of fear-based thinking—what we might call *low-vibration beliefs*. In contrast, feelings of connection, inspiration, and peace tend to arise when our thoughts are aligned with love, possibility, and self-worth.

At your core, you are already whole, already worthy of love and abundance. You don't need to earn that—it is the truth of your being. You are an expression of love and life itself. You already have access to a full stream of flowing energy. But over time, we've learned to place blocks in the way. We've built habits of self-doubt, fear, and resistance. These aren't who we are. They're just well-practised patterns.

The good news is: patterns can be changed. And it begins with a decision.

To trade fear for freedom, we must first identify the beliefs and behaviours that no longer serve us. Often, the behaviour made sense at one time—it served a purpose, met a need, helped us feel safe. Habits form to conserve energy; they become automatic shortcuts the brain uses to save effort. Like a groove in a well-worn path, the neural connection strengthens every time we repeat the thought or behaviour.

Think about learning to drive. The first time behind the wheel, you were likely hyper-aware—checking mirrors, judging pressure on pedals, nervous about every turn. There were so many things to remember, it felt overwhelming. But now? You drive without thinking. In fact, you might get home and not remember the drive at all. That's the power—and the danger—of habit.

Along the way, you may have also picked up some bad habits. Maybe you eat, text, or reach into the back seat while driving. These behaviours, like all habits, become automatic. And just like poor driving habits can damage a car, unconscious mental habits can derail a life.

That's why now is the perfect time to review the early conclusions you formed as a child. It's time to challenge those old beliefs and assumptions and replace them with conscious decisions. When you shift from *"This is just who I am"* to *"This is something I can change"*, you take back your power.

The brain may try to resist this. That's okay. Unfamiliar behaviours feel awkward at first. They require more effort—more energy, more attention. It's like taking a new route home. You notice everything: the road, the signs, the turns. You might feel excited. Or nervous. Maybe even exhausted by the end. But the awareness is sharper—and with repetition, the unfamiliar becomes familiar.

New neural pathways begin to form. With time, they strengthen. The effort fades. The path becomes smoother.

Creating new habits of thought and behaviour—ones rooted in love, self-worth, and presence—takes intention. It may involve journaling, therapy, breathwork, meditation, affirmations, or simply pausing long enough to reframe your inner dialogue. Whatever tools resonate with you, the key is this: stay committed. Be compassionate. And keep nurturing your growth like you would a seedling. It needs attention. It needs care. But it *will* grow.

Yes, releasing old beliefs takes energy. But holding onto them takes even more.

You are not broken. You are not your habits. You are not your past beliefs.

You are the one who is aware.

You are the one who can choose again.

And from that place of choice, transformation begins.

Knowing what needs to change is one thing. Doing it is another. The truth is, we don't have forever. There comes a moment when reflection must become action.

NO MORE WAITING – IT'S NOW

As a former nurse, I've witnessed my fair share of loss. One experience, in particular, has never left me. I was working in the Neonatal Intensive Care Unit—caring for a very sick, premature baby girl. She was born at 28 weeks gestation, her body so tiny and her systems so underdeveloped that life outside the womb was a constant battle. Despite months of medical support and the tireless care of her family and our team, she eventually lost her fight.

It was devastating. Not only for her family, but for many of us nurses who had come to know and love them. We didn't always attend the hospital chapel services, but I remember that one vividly. The small white coffin, barely the size of a pillow, held not just the body of a tiny soul—but also the quiet echo of a life that had come and gone too soon. That moment left an imprint on my heart and soul. It reminded me, in the most confronting way, just how fragile and fleeting life is.

Whether death is expected or sudden, it brings with it a wave of shock, grief, and often, a re-evaluation of what really matters. I am deeply grateful that both my parents and all my siblings are still here. And yet, I'm aware that every day is a gift we're not guaranteed.

There have been times—when I'm stressed, short-tempered, or just caught up in the busy-ness of life—where I've had to stop myself and ask: *"If this moment were the last one I ever had with them, what would I wish I'd said or done differently?"* In those moments of reactivity—when I feel myself pulling away or shutting down—I try to soften. To lean in rather than lash out. Because one day, I won't have that chance. And when that day comes, I want to know I chose love more often than not.

Too often, it takes a catastrophic event to wake us up. But we don't need to wait for tragedy to remember what's important. We can begin right now—by choosing to live with intention, appreciation, and presence. To say the things we mean. To show people we love them. To live a life that reflects our values. A life that we're proud of.

To be human is to feel the full spectrum of emotion—grief and joy, love and fear, heartbreak and hope. But beneath all of it is something deeper: the soul's longing to shine through. I believe we each carry a spark of inspired purpose. A quiet knowing that we are here to make a difference. And yet, so often, it is fear—not fate—that keeps us from moving forward. Fear of failure. Fear of rejection. Fear of the unknown.

But our soul is calling us to expand beyond that. And we must decide which voice we will follow.

For me, prioritising health and wellbeing is not just a value—it's a necessity. Without it, I don't get to experience this life, love my people, or fulfil my purpose. I teach my family this too: your health is your greatest investment. It's the foundation upon which everything else rests.

That said, I'm still growing. I'm still learning. I'm still working through old patterns and striving to do better. Most of us are. And that's okay. What matters is our willingness to keep choosing growth—to step into who we really are and allow that authentic self to be seen and felt in the world.

You don't have to wait for a near-death experience or a life-altering event to wake up to what matters.

You can start right now.
With this breath.
With this choice.

Choose to be present. Choose to love openly. Choose to take care of yourself. Choose to act from your heart. Choose to notice the miracles in the mundane.

Every moment is a sacred invitation—no matter how ordinary it appears.

You can experience joy.
You can experience grief.
You can experience both—knowing they are not opposites, but companions on the same journey.

Moments are fleeting. Let them pass *through* you, not by you. Be with them. Feel them. Honour them. And then—when they pass—be ready for the next one. Because life is not waiting.

And neither should you.

When we begin to live this way—present, grateful, and open—we change the trajectory of our lives. And when we do, we discover something else: every ending holds the potential for something beautiful.

THERE'S ALWAYS A GOOD ENDING

Whatever you choose from here is entirely up to you—and it will be enough. There will be moments when fear and worry tint your lens, and others when love and joy feel as natural as breath. Neither is wrong. Life will invite you into both, but the more you practice returning to love, the more peace you'll experience. It takes intention. It takes presence. But it's worth it.

You are the author now. The rest of your story is yours to write. You get to decide how it unfolds—but you don't have to write it alone. You are part of a wider community. One that's waking up, showing up, and choosing to live from the heart. And your presence matters. You have the power to influence and inspire those around you, not by preaching or performing, but simply by being.

Every time you choose compassion over criticism…
Every time you pause instead of react…
Every time you come back to love instead of fear…
You create a ripple.

I've seen it happen in my own family. I've watched my clients reconnect with their own essence, and in doing so, change the energy of their homes, their workplaces, their friendships. Your presence has the potential to transform—not only your own life but the lives you touch.

So here's my invitation: if you're ready to keep living and growing in alignment with love, you're welcome to join a growing movement—a *FeelGood* community committed to living consciously, courageously, and joyfully.

Being part of something bigger helps you stay grounded in your intention. It's easy to drift. But with support, it's also easier to return. You don't need to have it all figured out—just a willingness to keep coming back to what matters most.

One day, my own journey will come full circle. I'll look back and feel immense gratitude for the life I've lived. I hope there are still many years ahead to create, love, and grow. And I hope the same for my family, my friends, and for you—the reader who's walked beside me through these pages.

I trust, with certainty, that all will be well.

As for my son, whose early health challenges once cast a shadow over our dreams—I recently watched him receive his tapping teacher's certificate. A young student looked up at him and addressed him as "Mister". I smiled quietly, my heart full of joy.

In that simple moment, I knew: all was good in the world.

Yes, there is always a good ending. And the best part?
You get to create it.

The ending of a book is often seen as the closing of something. But this is not that kind of ending.

This is a living, breathing invitation. A doorway, not a finish line. You are not who you were when you began this journey. You've reflected. You've paused. You've challenged beliefs and rewired the inner workings of your story. And now, you walk forward more awake.

There is no single moment that marks the end of becoming—only moments of deeper alignment, fuller embodiment, and expanded love. Life will still challenge you. But now you meet it differently. You carry new awareness. A deeper compassion. A stronger trust in your inner knowing.

You've seen that the real problem was never "out there".
You've questioned the beliefs that shaped your limits.
You've remembered that the only real moment is now.
And you've discovered that the ending is always yours to create

So go ahead—live the story you want to tell.
Start from love.
Start from now.
And keep rewriting as you go.

There will be moments when you forget.
There will be days when the old stories call you back.
That's okay. You're not here to be flawless.
You're here to be fully human and fully awake—
Aware, compassionate, courageous enough to choose a new belief.

So choose.
Choose stillness when the world gets loud.
Choose love when fear tries to take the wheel.
Choose trust when the outcome is unknown.
Choose presence—again and again and again.

And if you ever feel alone, know this:
There is a community rising.
There are others—just like you—stepping into their own FeelGood truth.
Together, we are rewriting what it means to live a life of meaning.
Together, we're remembering the power that lives within us.
Together, we are the ripple.

I would be honoured to walk with you further.

You're warmly invited to connect with me in any of the following ways:

hello@denisemokadsi.com.au

www.denisemokadsi.com.au

www.linkedin.com/in/denisemokadsi/

Let this not be the closing of a book—
Let it be a reminder to believe your truth.

And if you ever forget…
Just come back to this:

You are love.
You are light.
You are enough.

Chapter Highlights

Seeing the Real Problem:
Real transformation begins by identifying the root cause beneath symptoms and behaviours.

Believe It. Or Not:
Our beliefs are often formed through childhood conditioning and go unquestioned into adulthood. Many limiting thoughts are based on assumptions, not truths—and can be rewritten.

No More Waiting – It's Now:
You are free to express your true self and live with purpose now—not someday.

There's Always a Good Ending:
There is always hope, healing, and beauty —even in the endings.

REFLECTIVE QUESTIONS

1. What "problem" in your life might actually be a symptom of something deeper?
   _____
   _____

2. What meaning have you attached to certain emotions or experiences that might need rewriting?
   _____
   _____

3. What empowering belief would you like to replace an old, limiting one with?
   _____
   _____

4. If today was your only day, what would you say or do differently?
   _____
   _____

5. How can you begin honouring your health, purpose, and relationships now—not later?
   _____
   _____

6. In what small ways can you be the ripple of love and healing for others today?
   _____
   _____

7. What does a "good ending" look and feel like for you—and what might be your next chapter?
   _____
   _____

THE BELIEF SHIFT

GRATITUDE AND ACKNOWLEDGEMENT

Thank you for walking this path with me.

No story is ever written alone.

This book may carry my voice, but it is filled with the echoes, encouragement, and wisdom of so many others.

To my family—thank you for being my greatest teachers.

To my sons: your resilience, humour, and light have inspired parts of this book I didn't even know were waiting to be written. Watching you both grow has been one of my life's most sacred joys.

To my husband: your love, patience, and quiet strength have grounded me through every rewrite, every doubt, and every breakthrough. You are my safe place to land, always.

To my parents and siblings: thank you for your presence in my life. Our shared history has helped shape my journey, and I honour both the beauty and the lessons.

To my clients and community: you are brave, heart-led souls. It is an honour to walk beside you. Your stories, your vulnerability, and your willingness to do the work have deeply informed these pages.

To my teachers, mentors, and guides (both formal and informal): your words, your challenges, and your faith in human potential have helped me find mine. I carry your influence with deep respect.

To my book coach Andrew Jobling: thank you for your belief in me as an author. This book would never have come to life if not for your words of encouragement and continued support throughout the writing process.

To my publisher Morpheus Publishing: thank you for helping me share the words of my thoughts with the world.

To my early readers, editors, and sounding boards: thank you for your thoughtful insights, your encouragement, and your generous time. This book is stronger because of you.

To the women navigating midlife, transformation, healing, and self-discovery: I see you. This book was written for you, with you, and because of you.

To Life itself: thank you for the beauty and the mess, the questions and the quiet answers. Thank you for the reminder that we are always evolving, always returning to love.

And finally, to *you*, the reader: thank you.

Thank you for showing up with an open heart.

Thank you for your willingness to reflect, to feel, to remember who you are and shift limiting beliefs to new empowering ones.

I hope these pages provided you not just insight, but also a felt sense of comfort, courage, and clarity.

May you continue to write your story with love.

With heartfelt appreciation,

Denise Mokadsi

www.ingramcontent.com/pod-product-compliance
Lightning Source LLC
Chambersburg PA
CBHW061207070526
44583CB00025B/3154